MYSTIC & BOYSEN

Go to the Dentist

Written by **Kimberly Griffiths**
Illustrated by **Lydia Wharton**

Mystic and Boysen Go to the Dentist
© Copyright Kimberly Griffiths 2019 First Edition
First Published in the USA by Spotlight Publishing, Goodyear AZ

ISBN: 978-1-7337388-8-0 Hardcover
ISBN: 978-1-7334077-0-0 Paperback
ISBN: 978-1-7337388-9-7 ebook

Library of Congress Cataloging-in-Publication Data: 2019910701

Cover: Jeremy Jimson
Illustrations by: Lydia Wharton
Book design: by Jeremy Jimson
Interior Layout: Becky Norwood

- Kimberly Griffiths
Mystic and Boysen Go to the Dentist

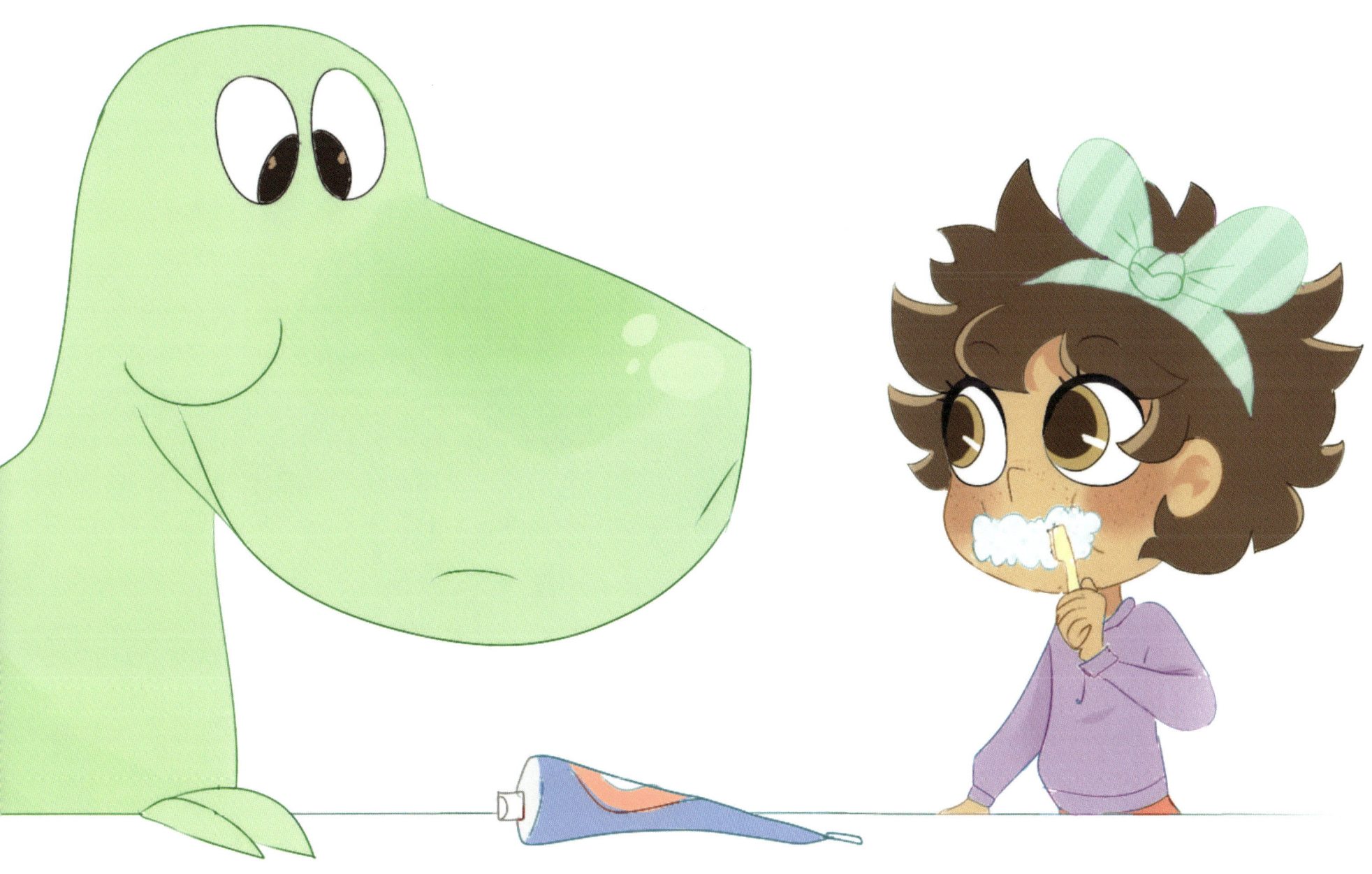

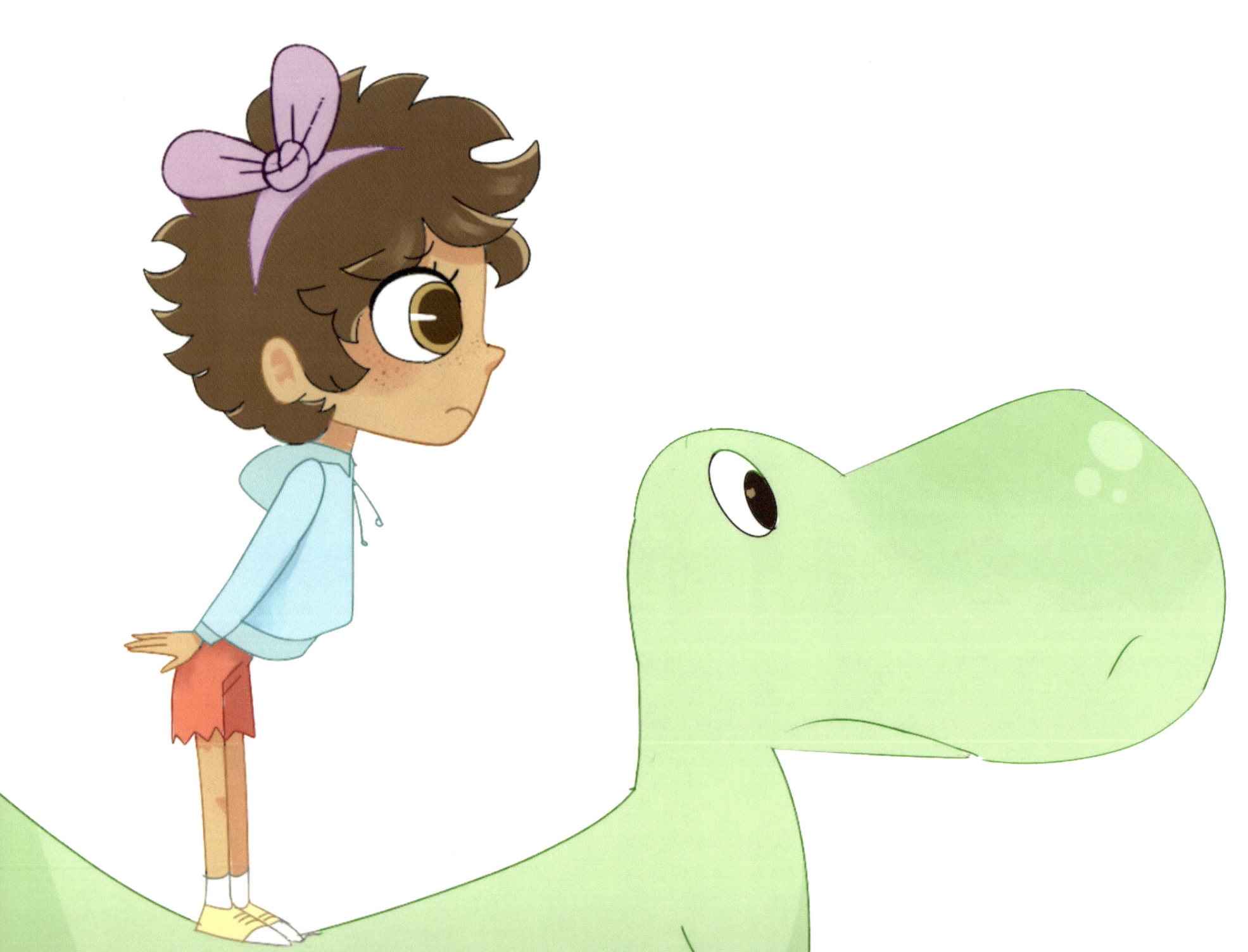

For Mom & Howie

For Sydney, Brian & the
Lhasa Apsos, who all inspire me

To Roberta, who said,
"Just write it!"

To Mom, Dad, Cleo & Toula,
Love, Lydia

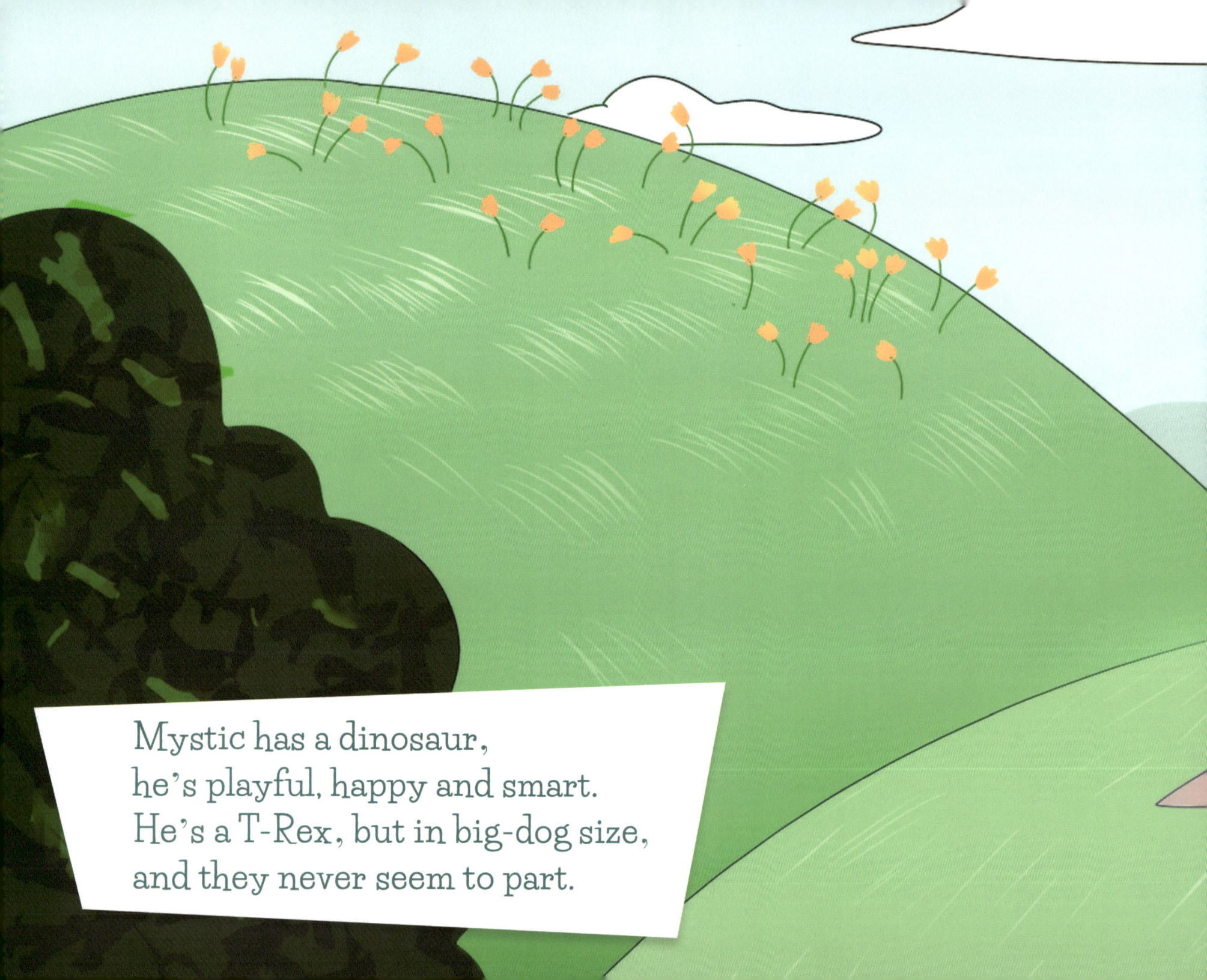

Mystic has a dinosaur,
he's playful, happy and smart.
He's a T-Rex, but in big-dog size,
and they never seem to part.

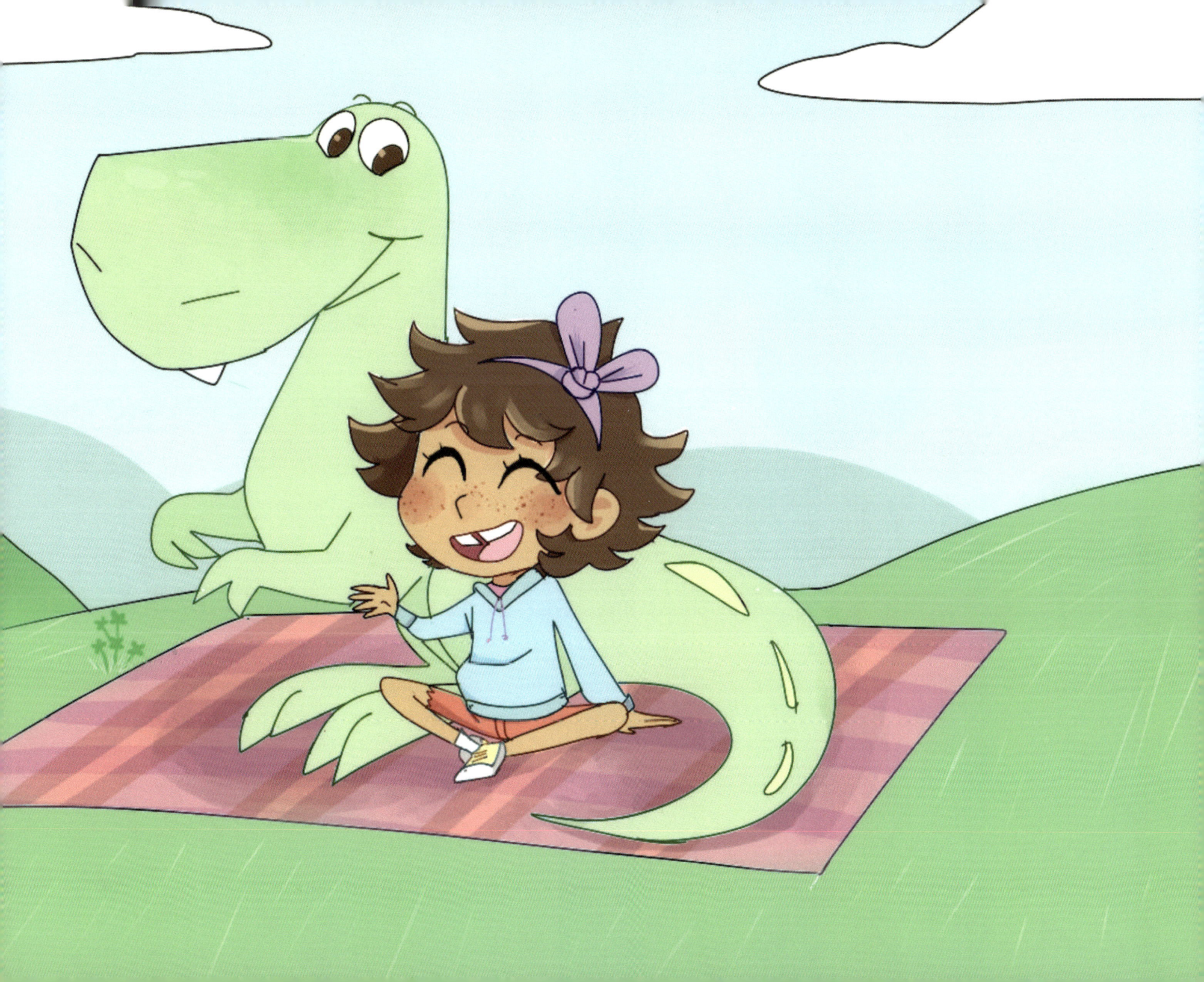

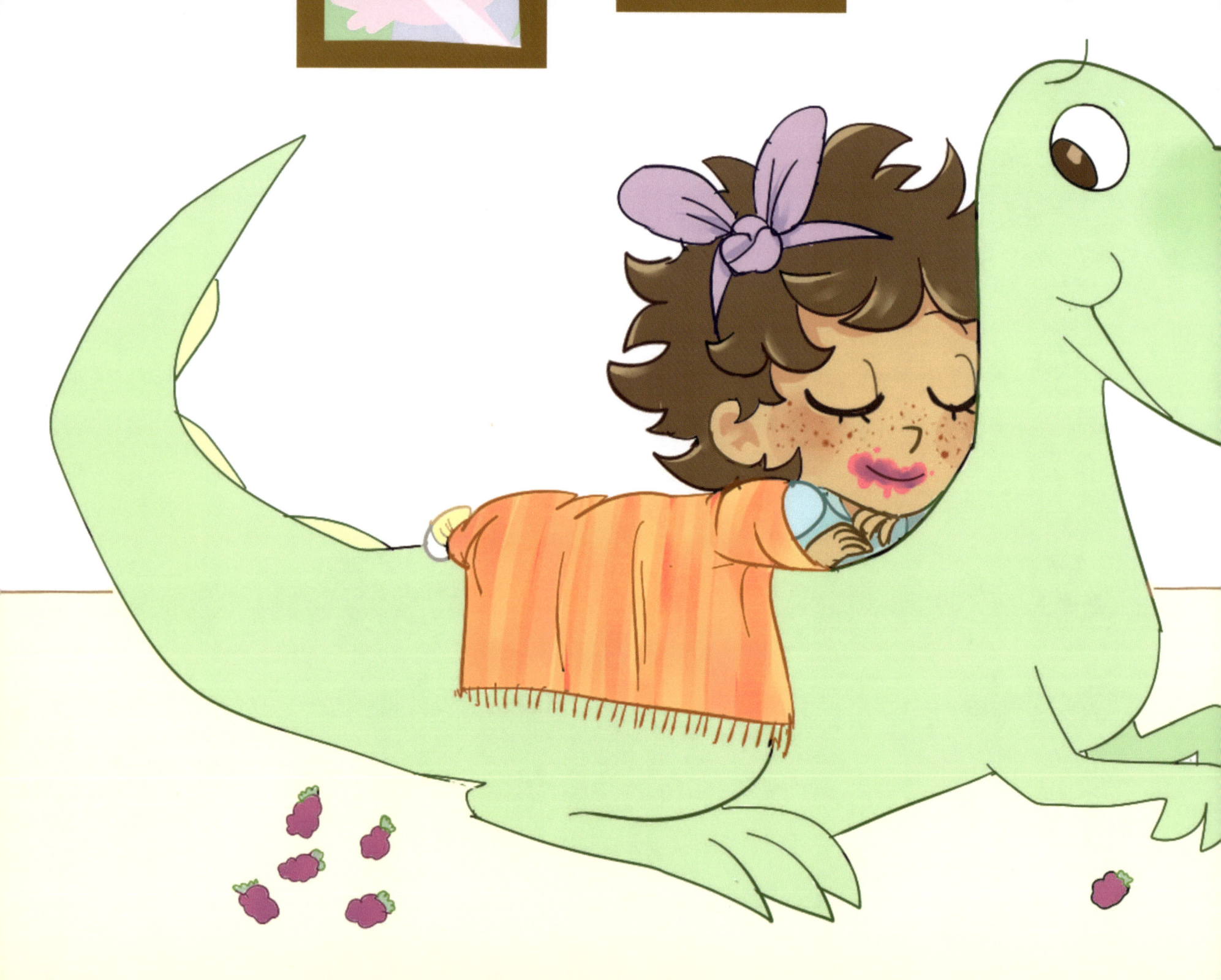

The dino's name is Boysen,
'Cuz that berry is Mystic's fave.
He's a friend and a brother all in one,
There's nothing they can't brave.

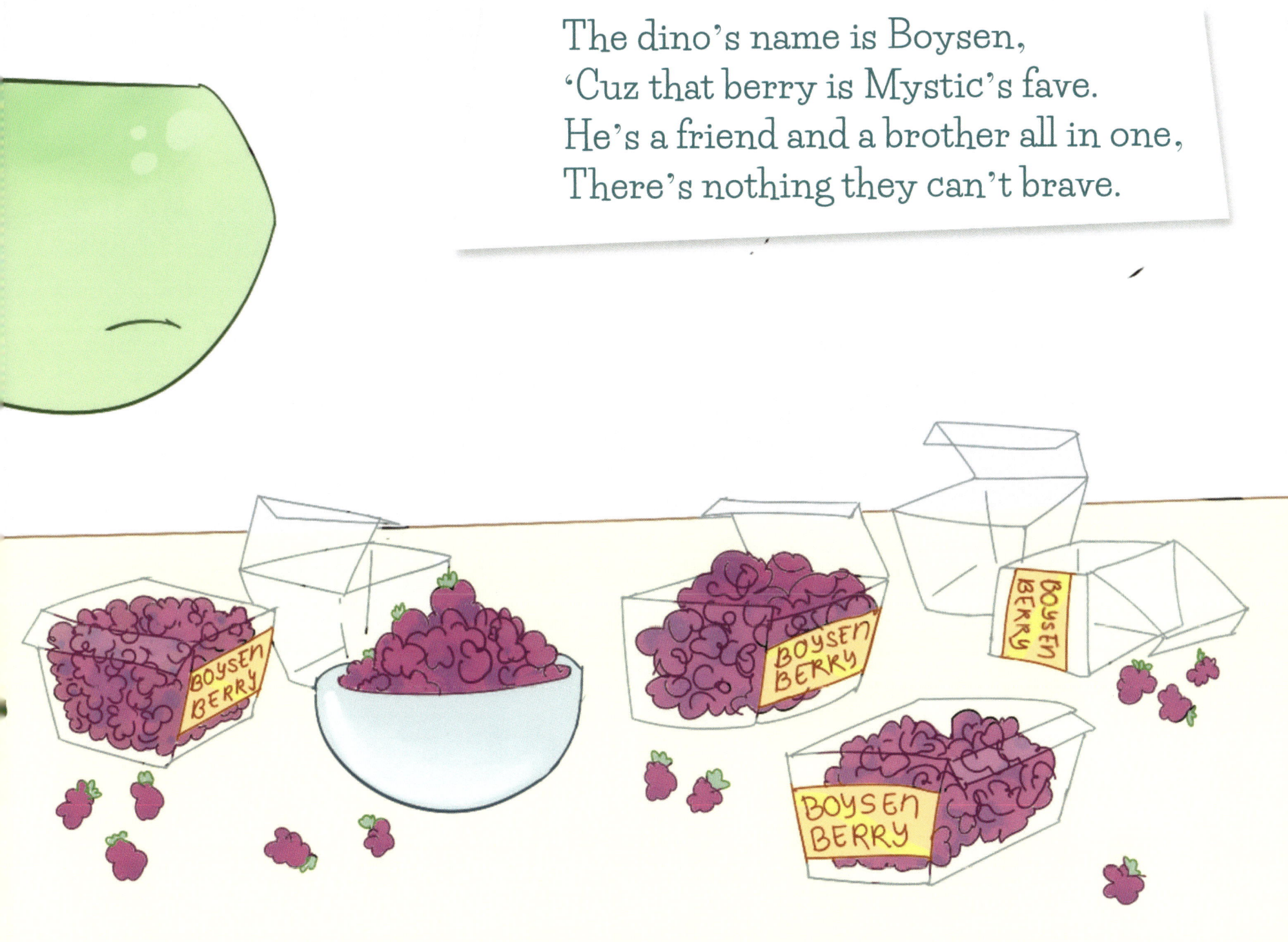

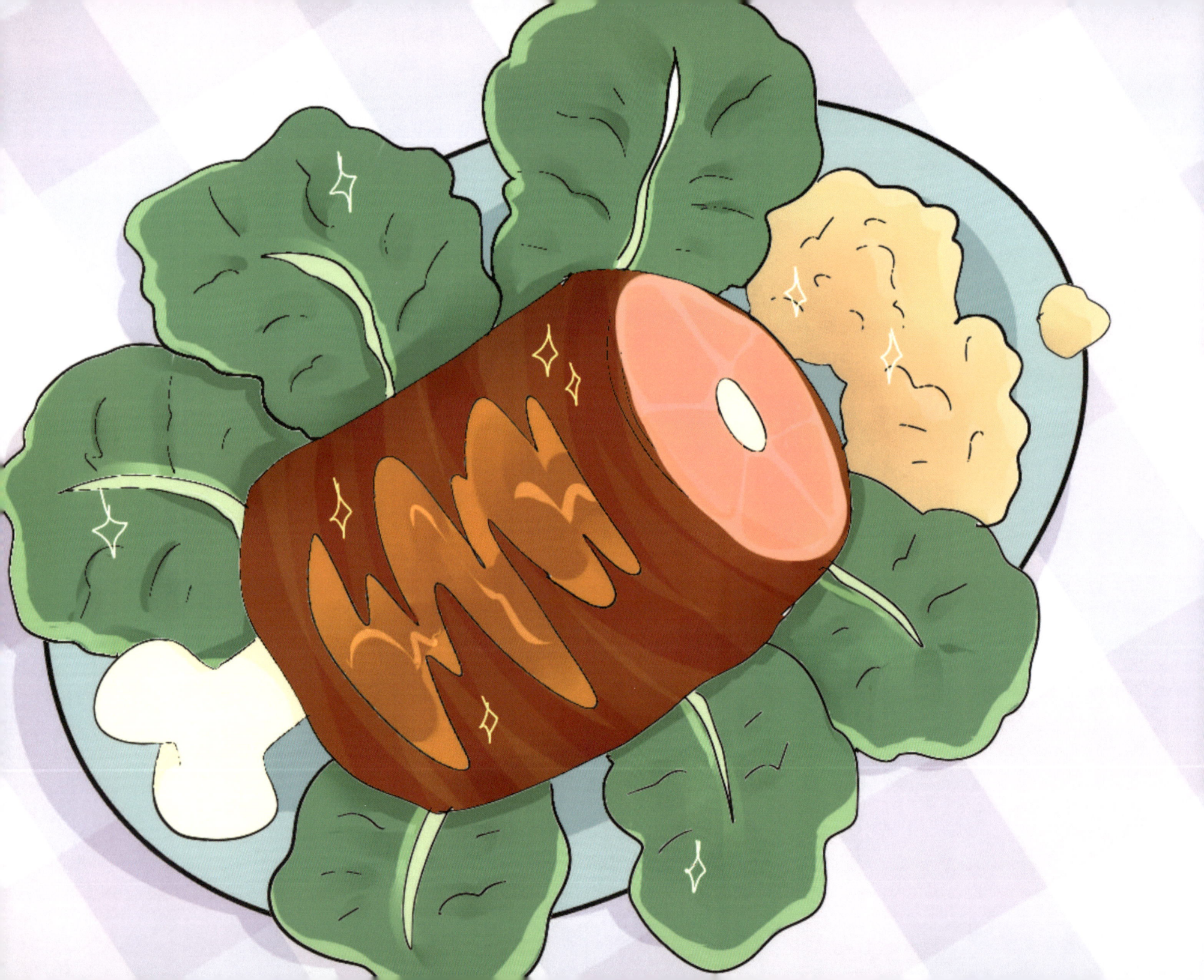

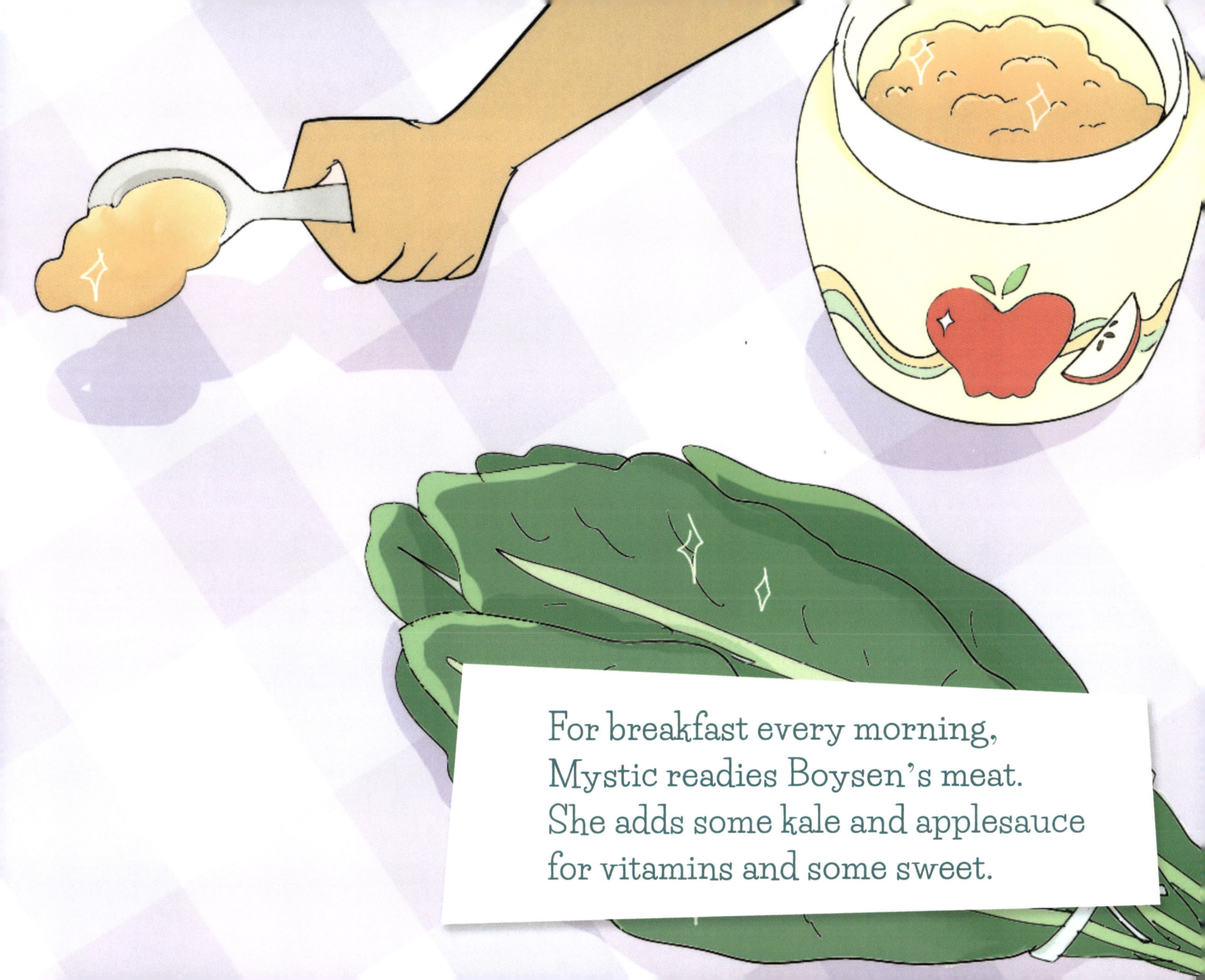

For breakfast every morning,
Mystic readies Boysen's meat.
She adds some kale and applesauce
for vitamins and some sweet.

On a beautiful, bright, spring day,
Mystic noticed sadly
that Boysen didn't want to chew.
He tried to hide it, but badly.

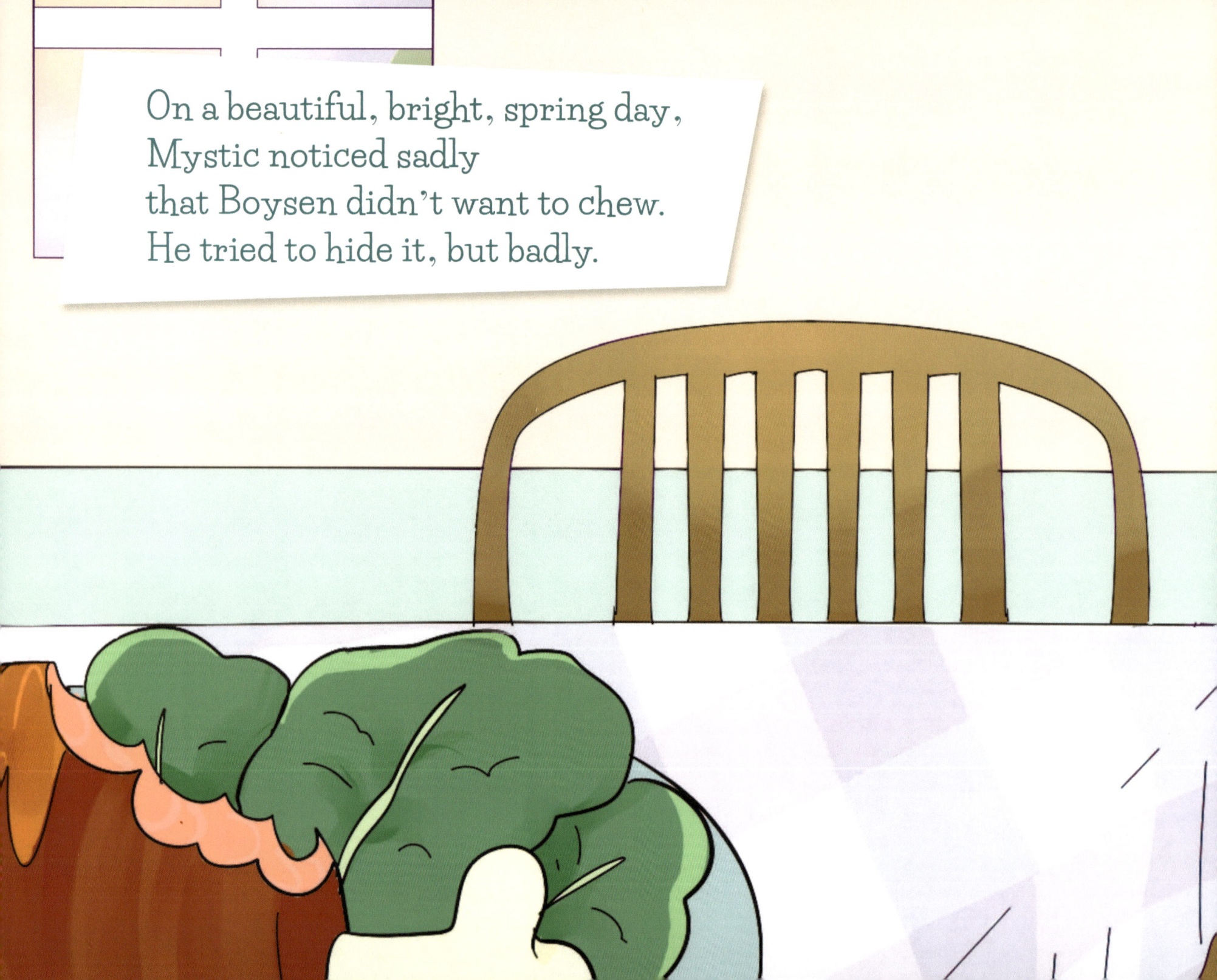

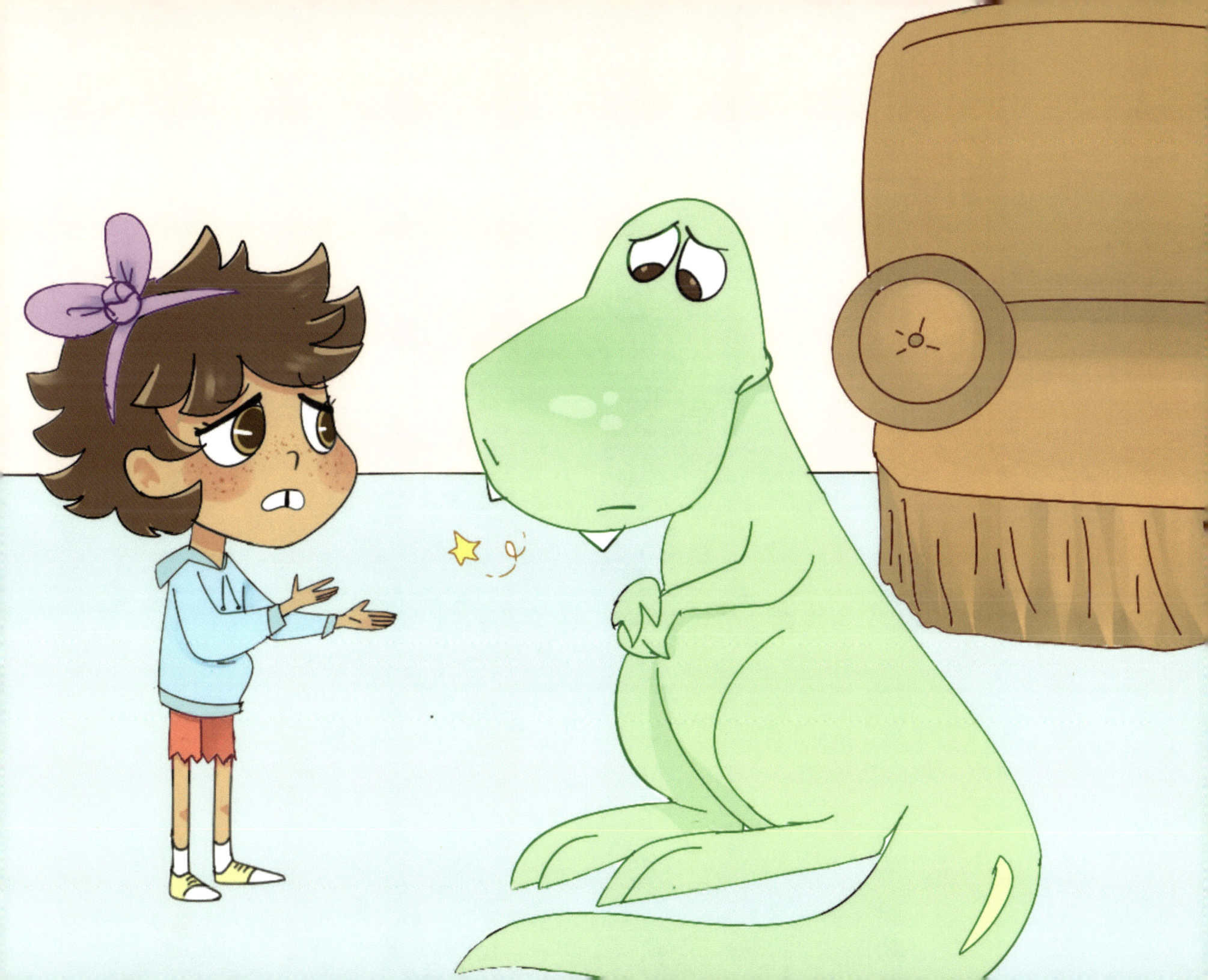

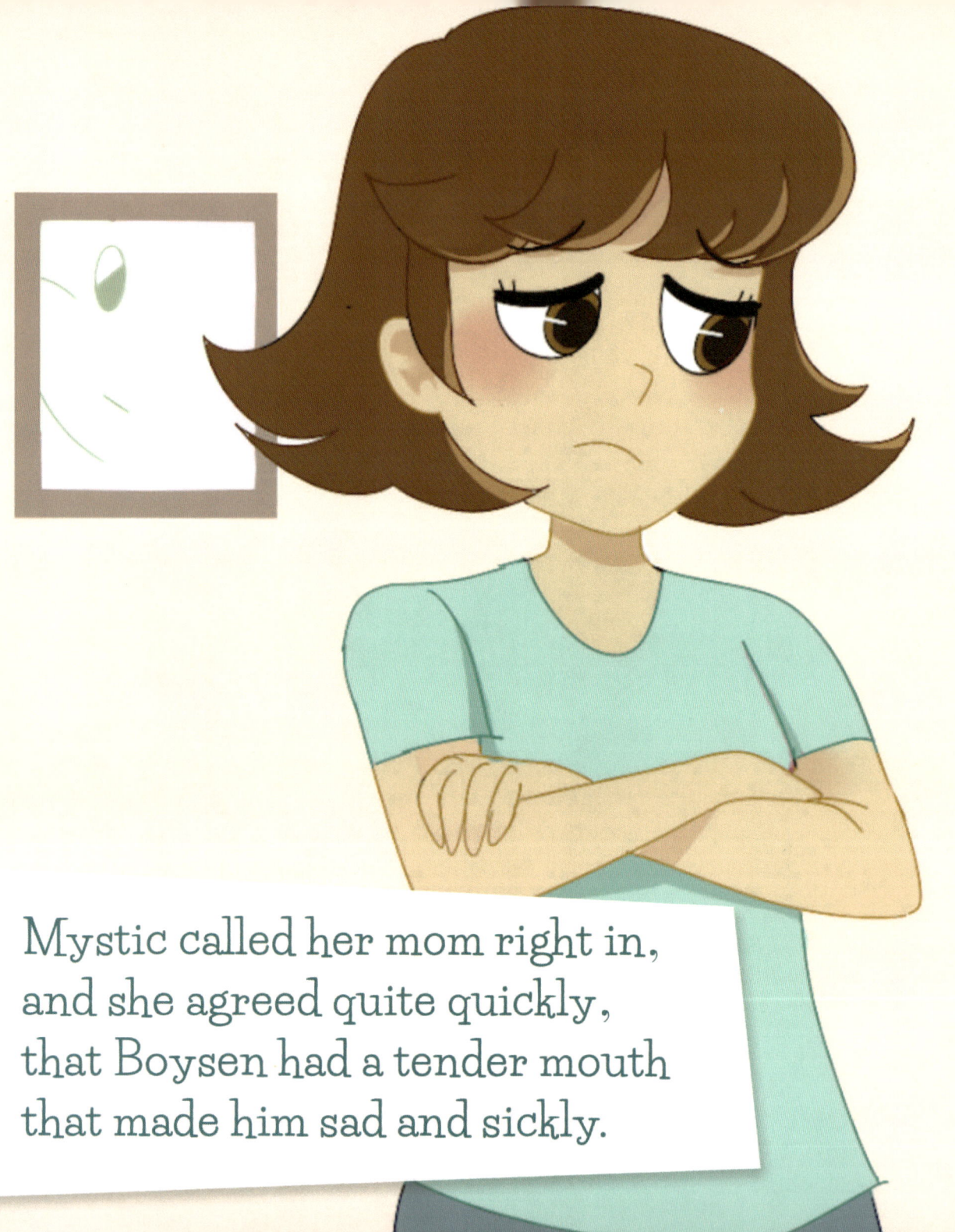

Mystic called her mom right in,
and she agreed quite quickly,
that Boysen had a tender mouth
that made him sad and sickly.

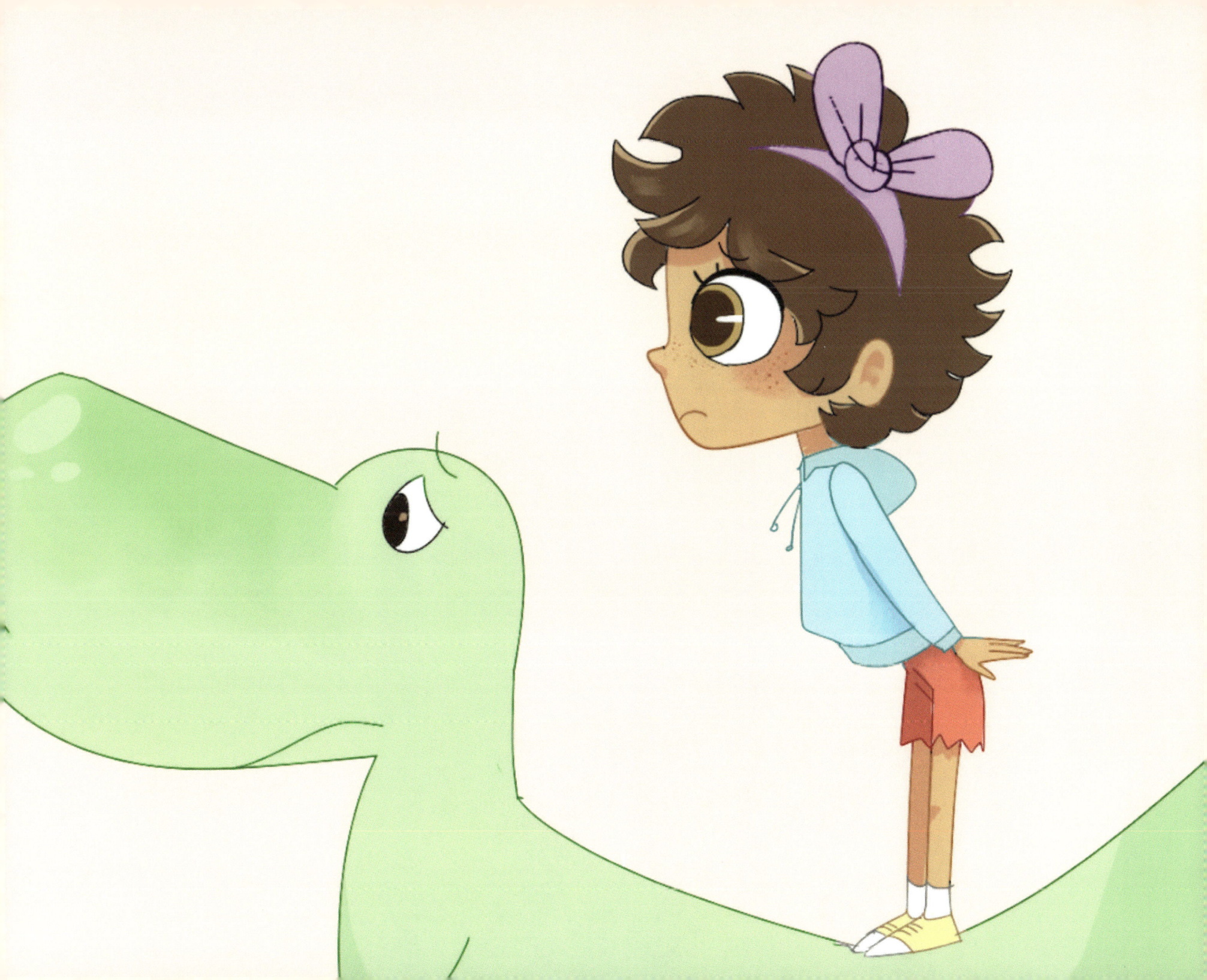

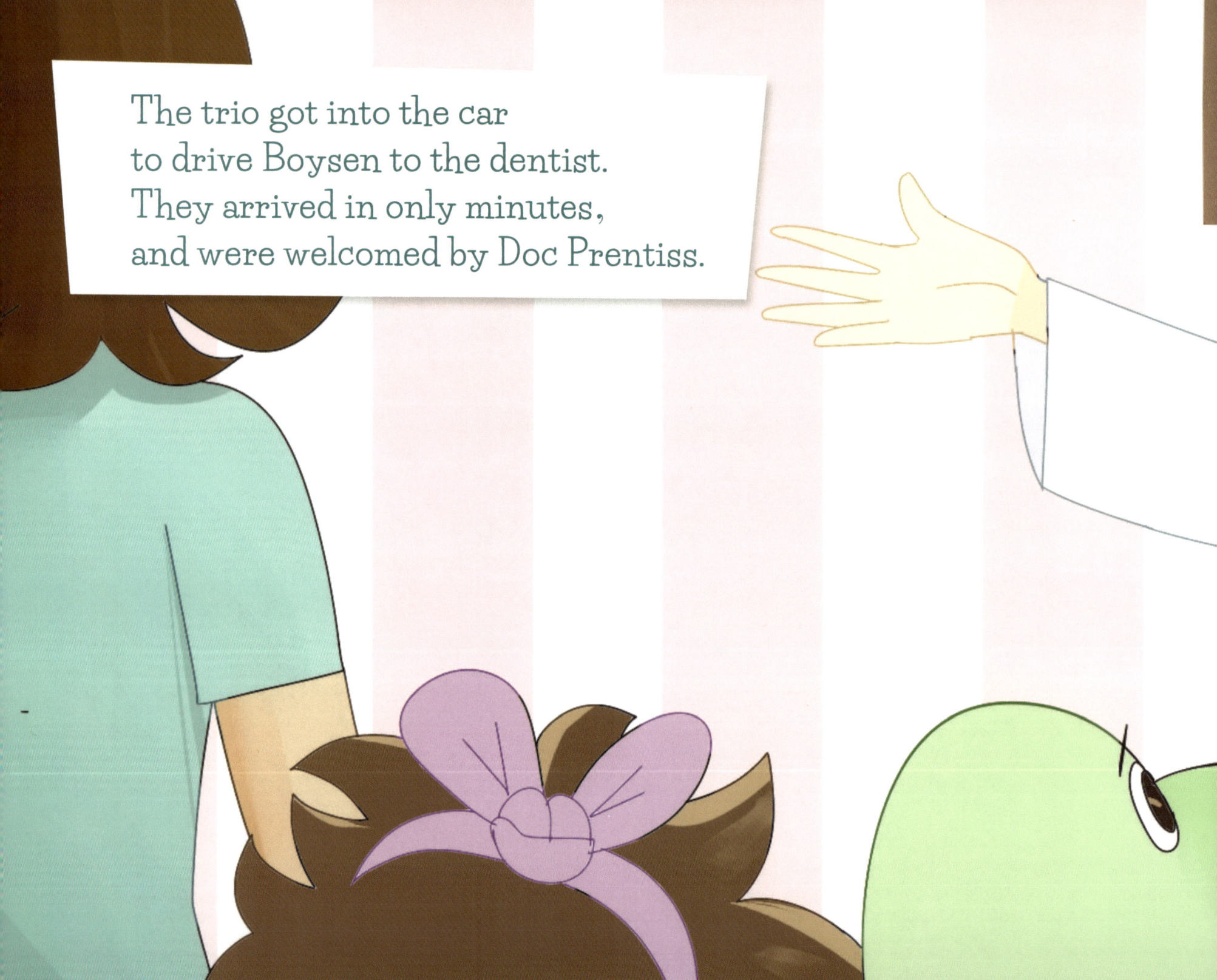

The trio got into the car
to drive Boysen to the dentist.
They arrived in only minutes,
and were welcomed by Doc Prentiss.

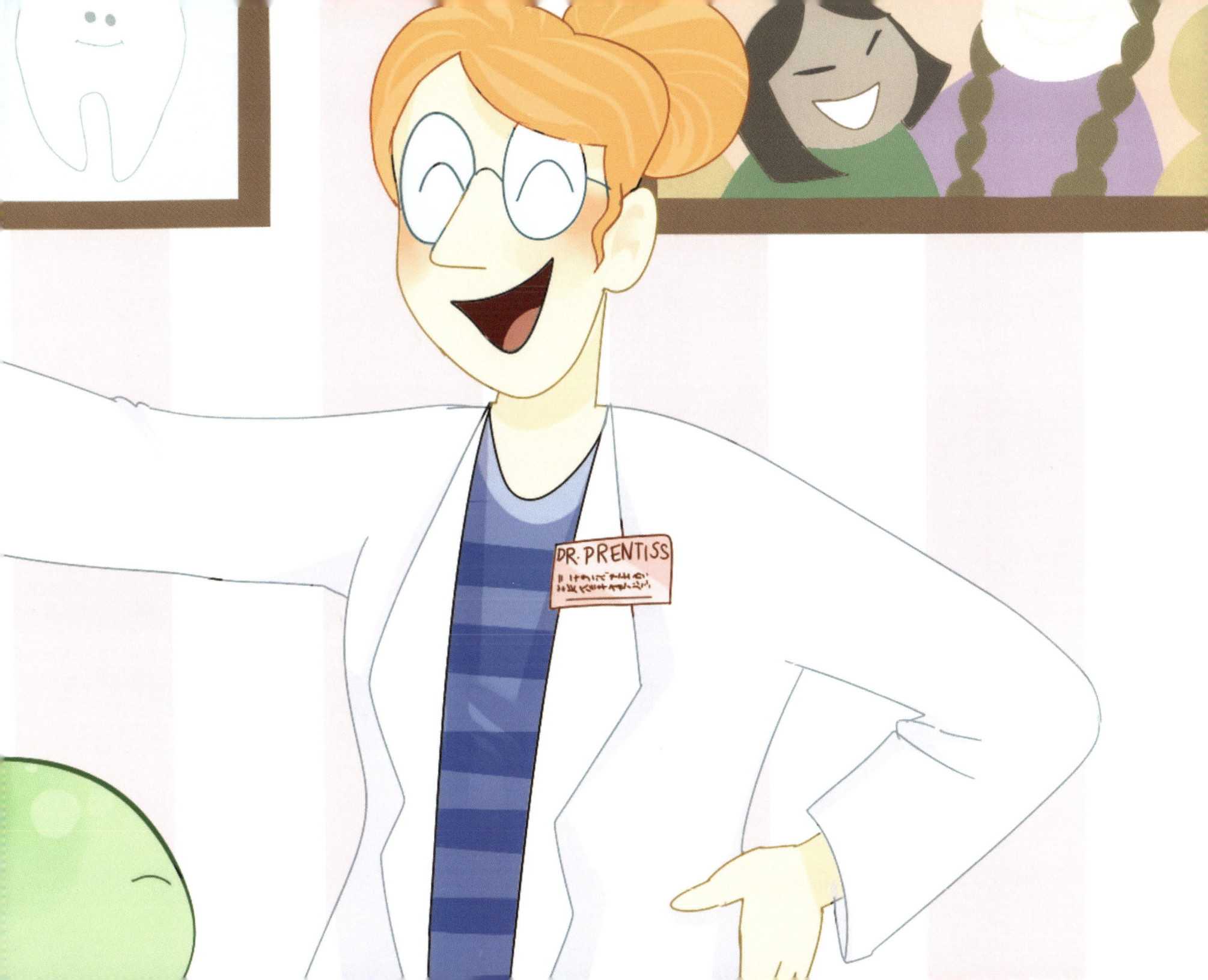

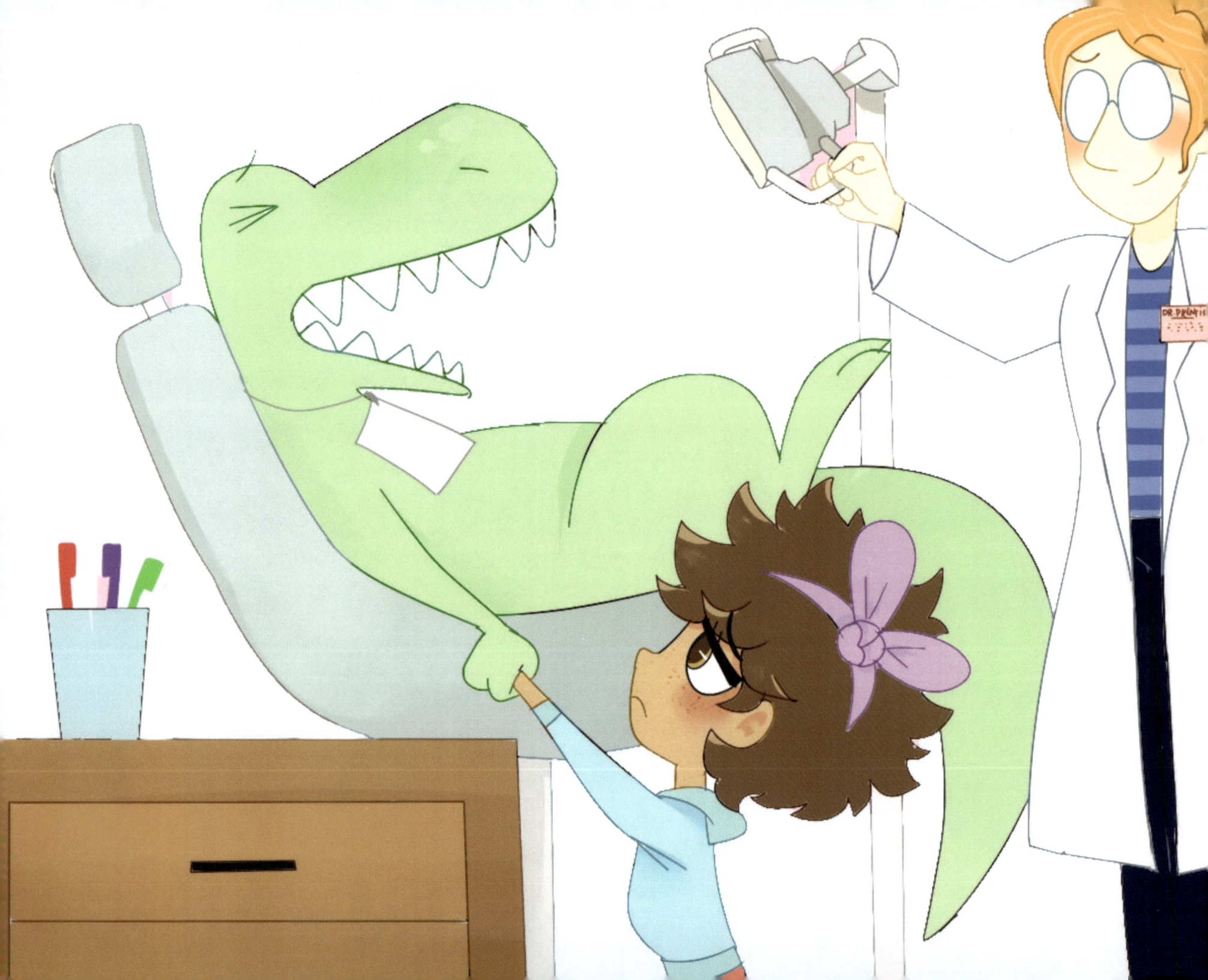

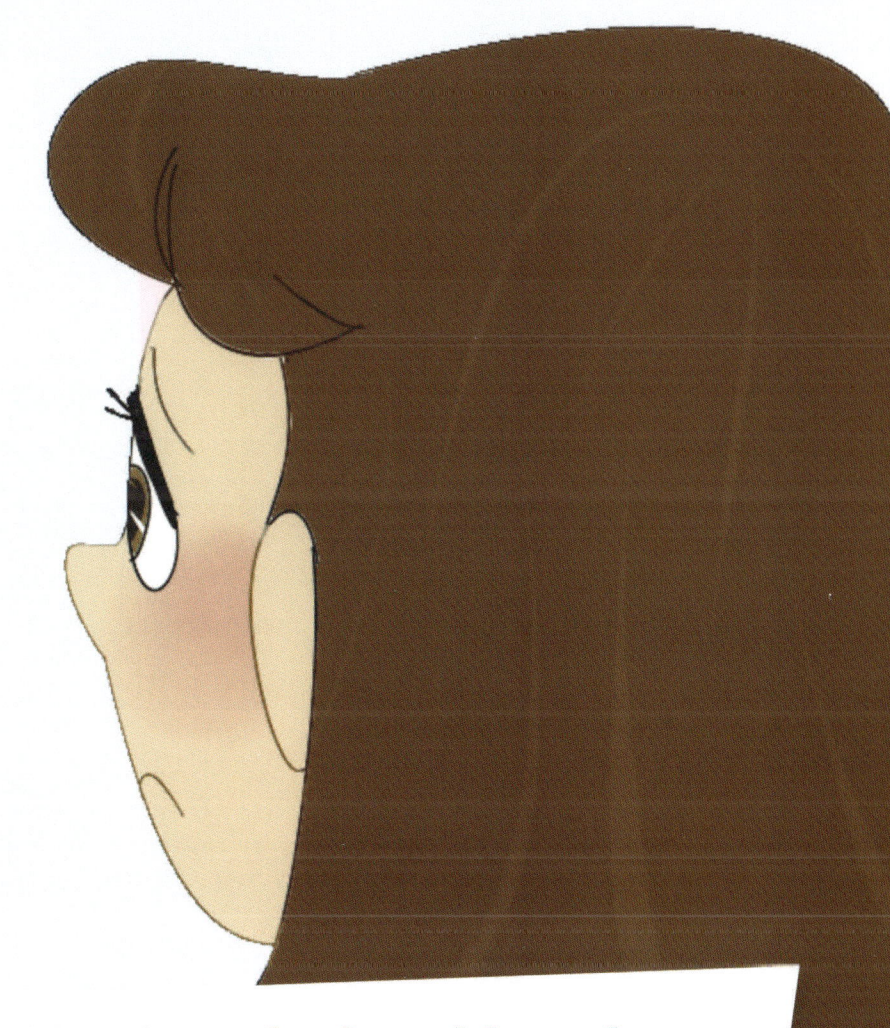

Boysen leaned back in the big, blue chair
holding Mystic's hand so tightly.
The doctor turned her spotlight on
lighting Boysen's jaws quite brightly.

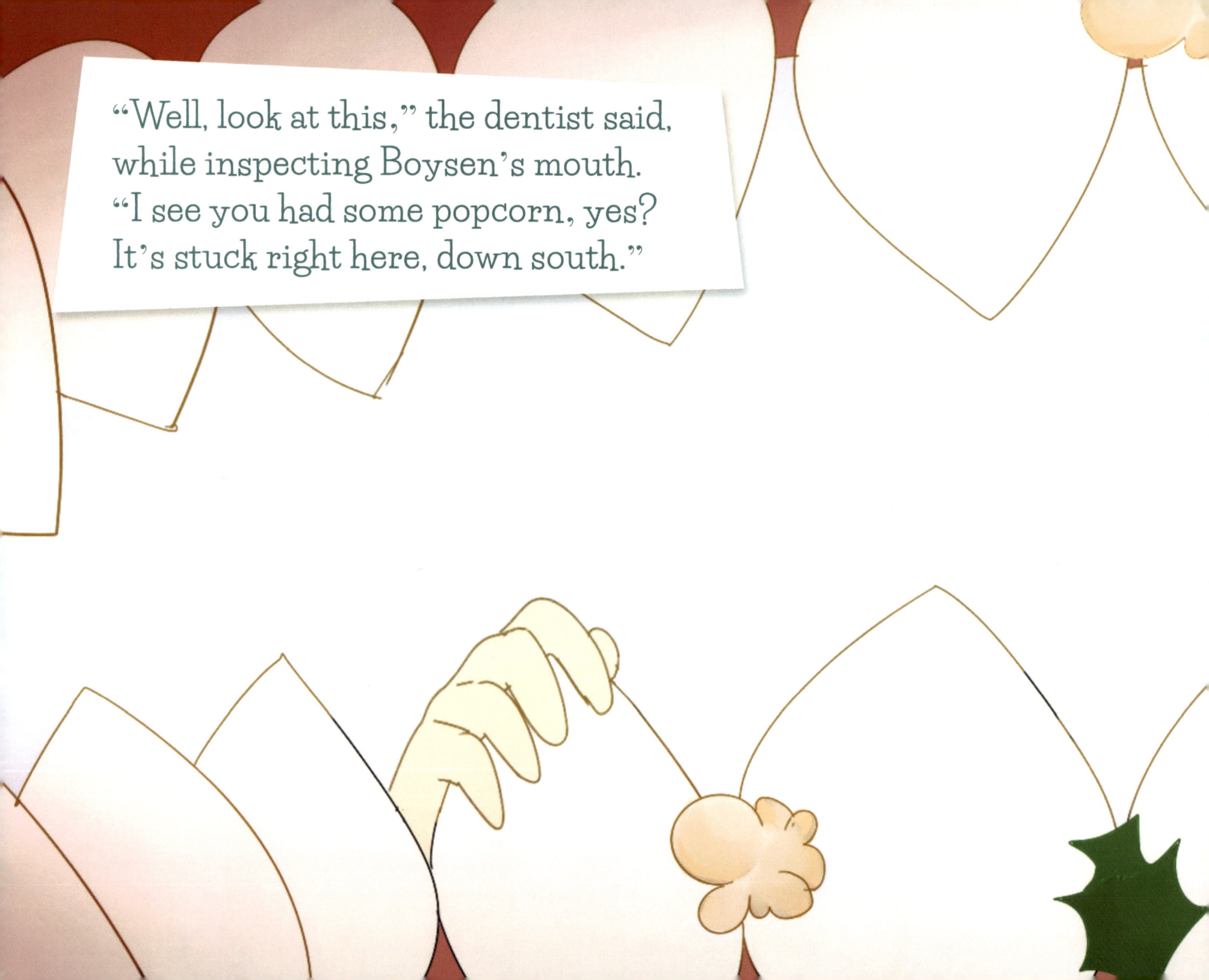

"Well, look at this," the dentist said,
while inspecting Boysen's mouth.
"I see you had some popcorn, yes?
It's stuck right here, down south."

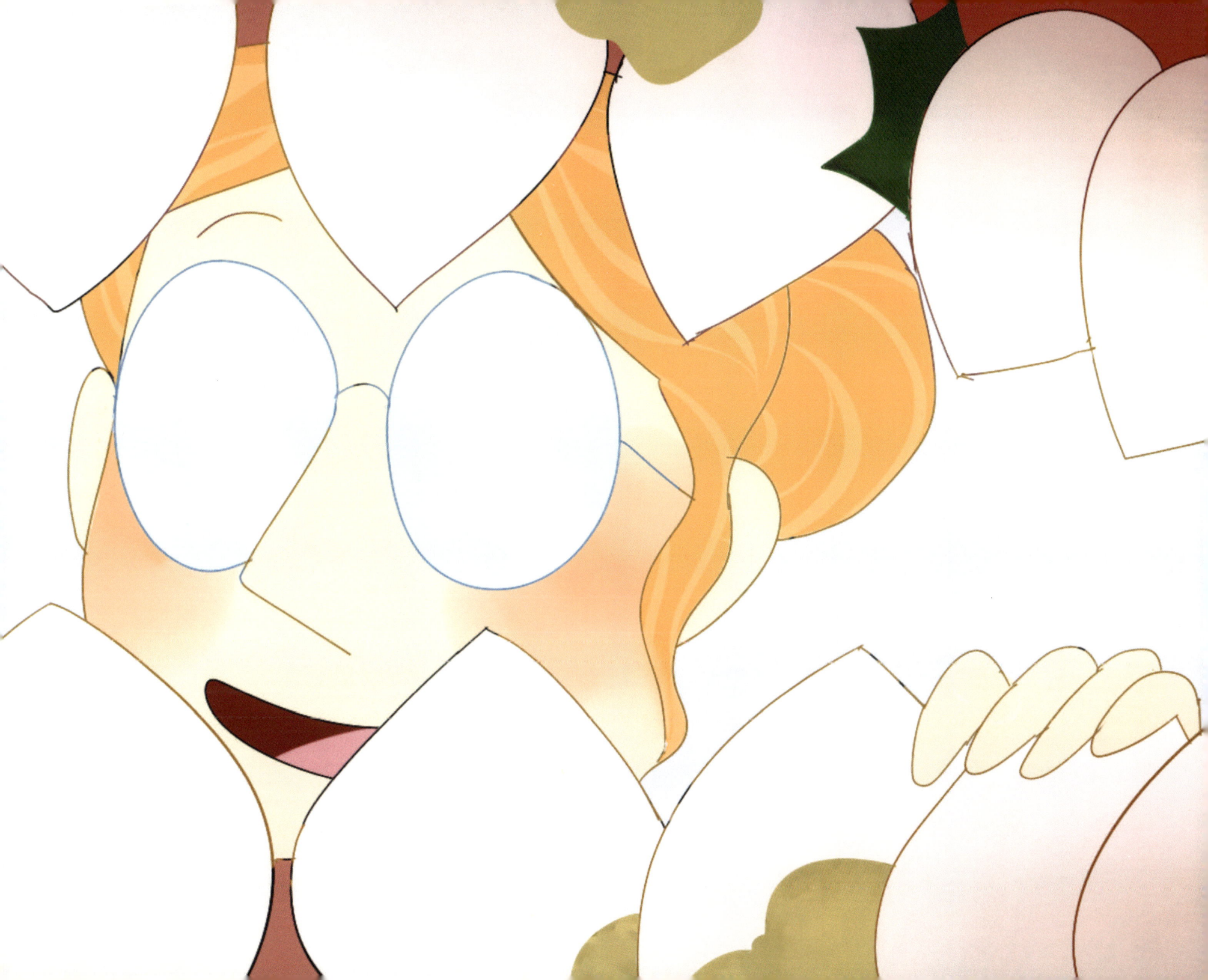

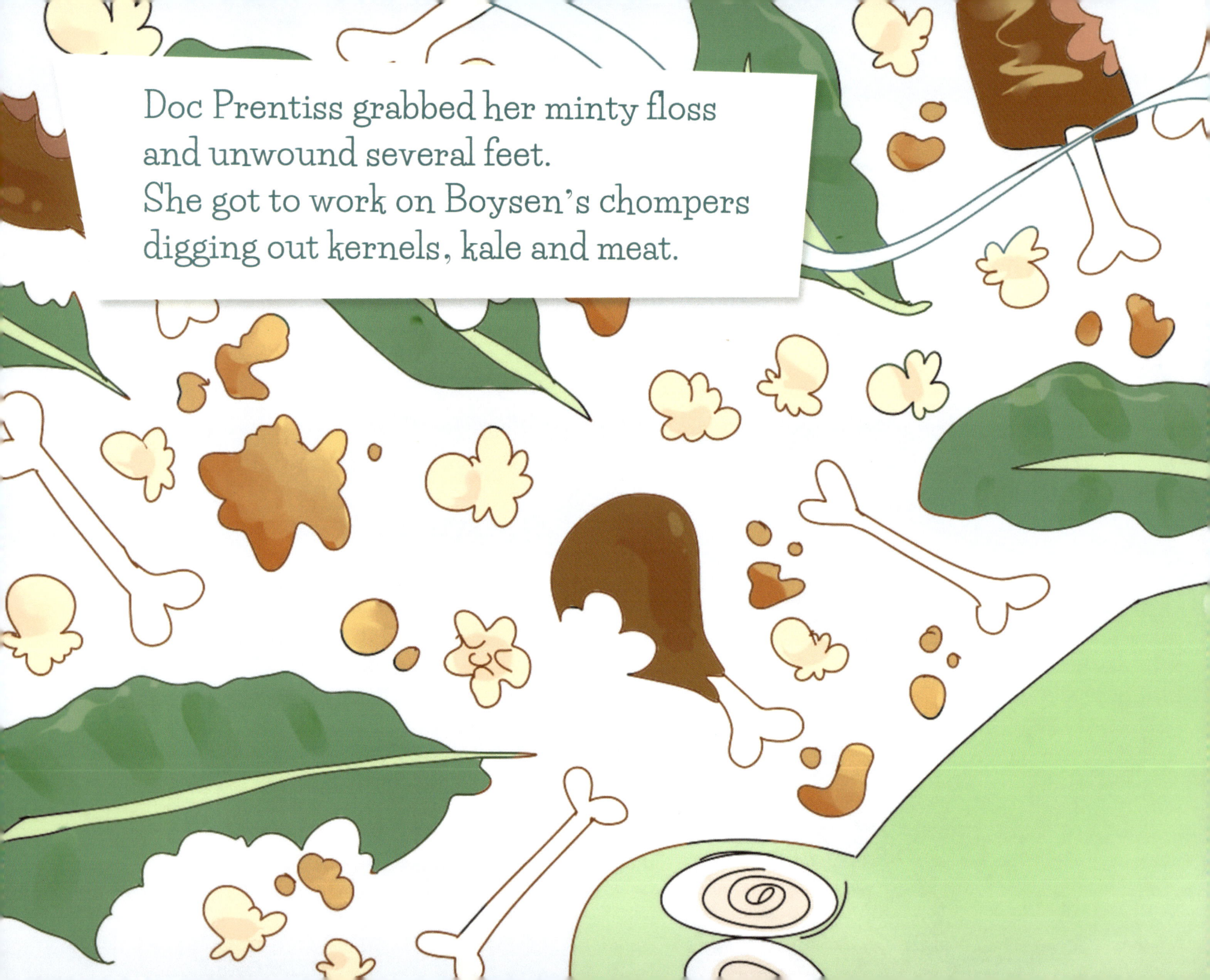

Doc Prentiss grabbed her minty floss
and unwound several feet.
She got to work on Boysen's chompers
digging out kernels, kale and meat.

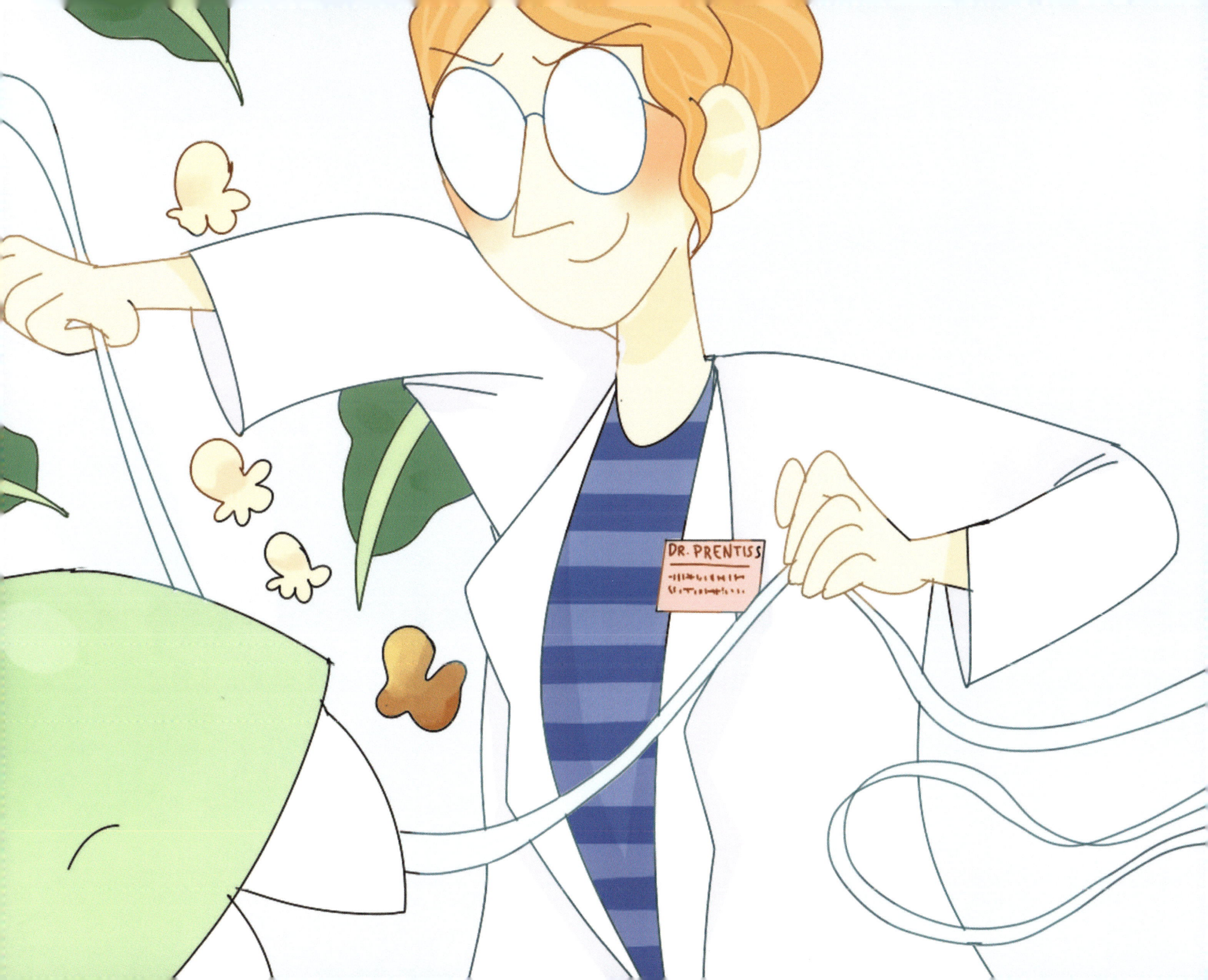

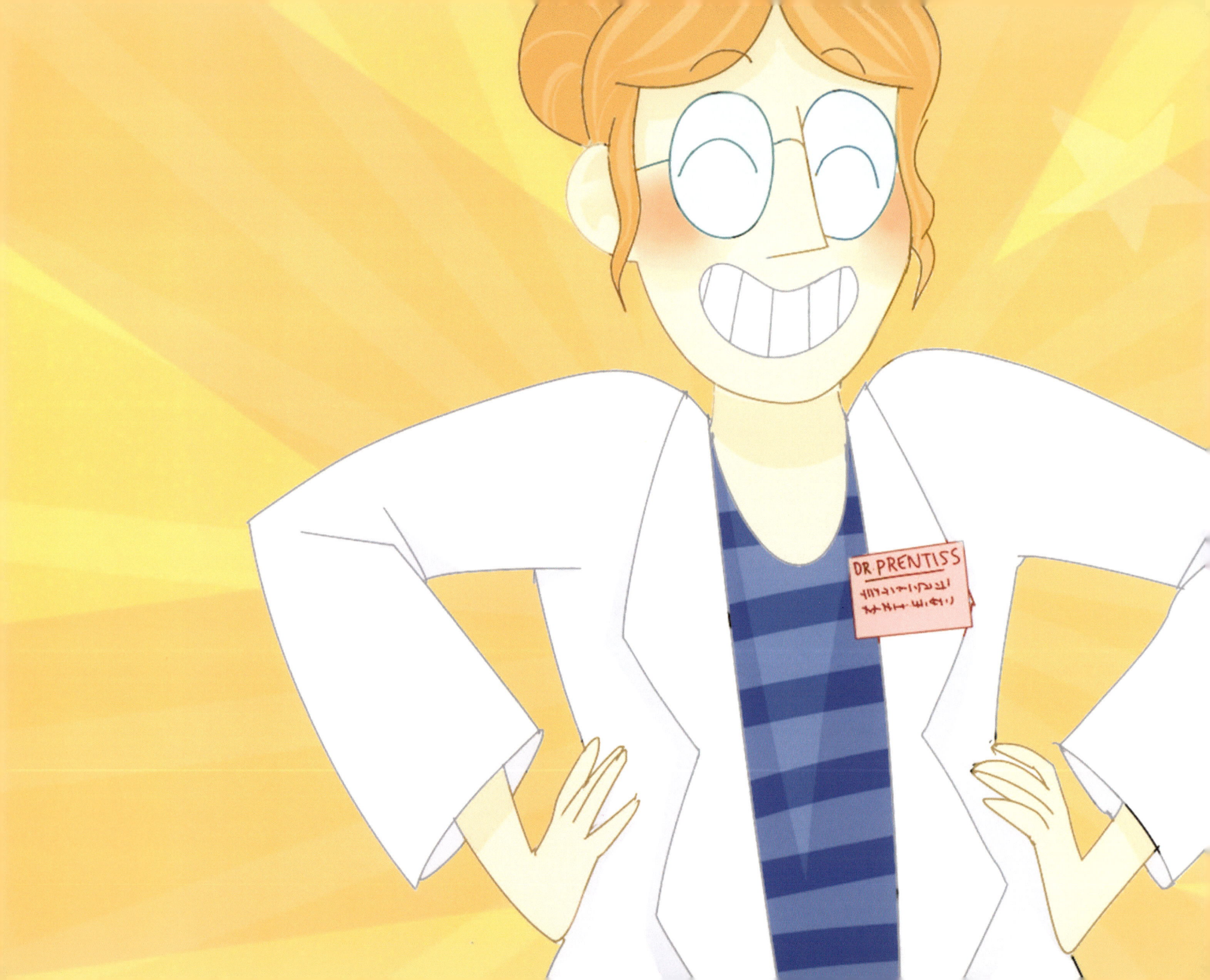

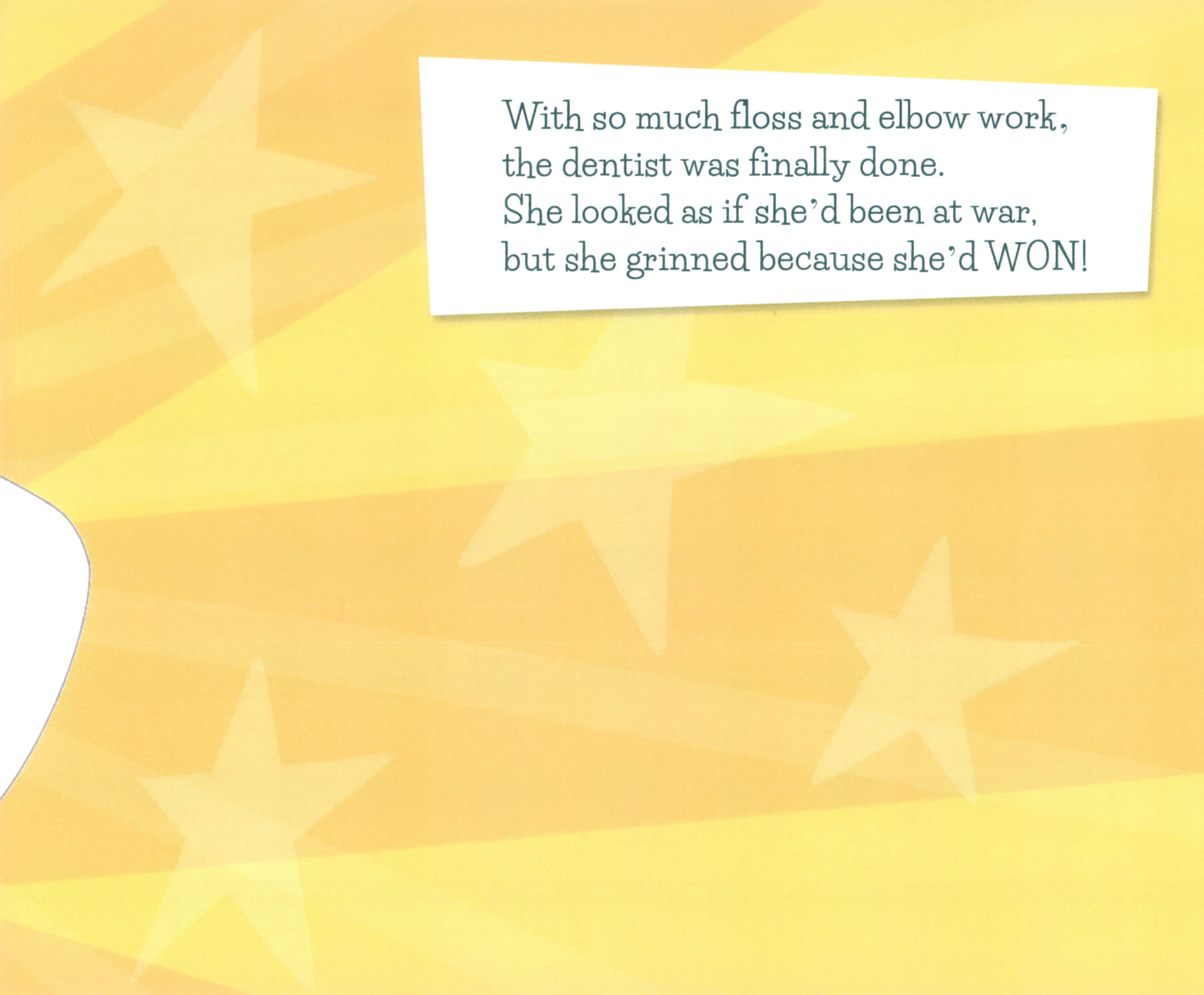

With so much floss and elbow work,
the dentist was finally done.
She looked as if she'd been at war,
but she grinned because she'd WON!

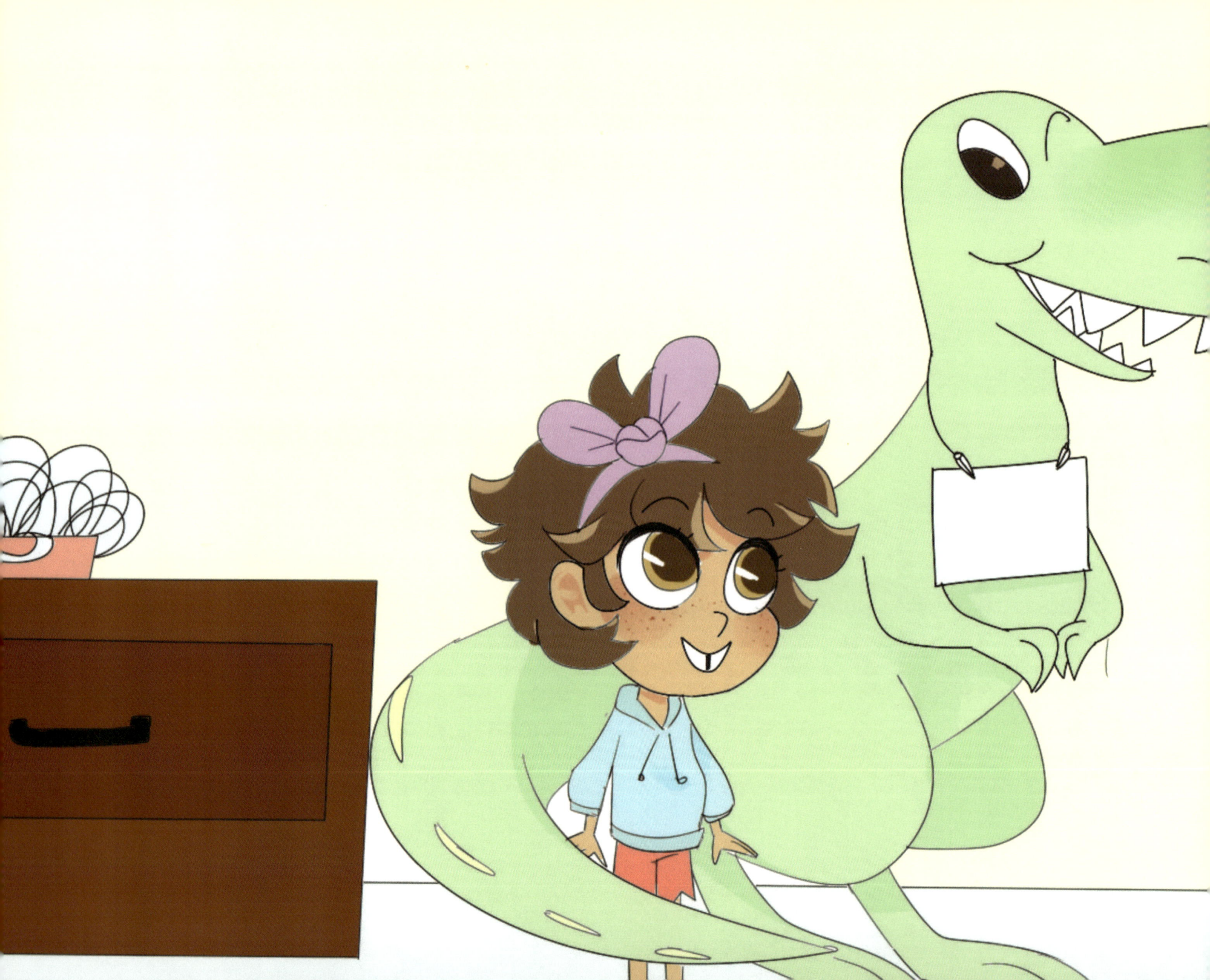

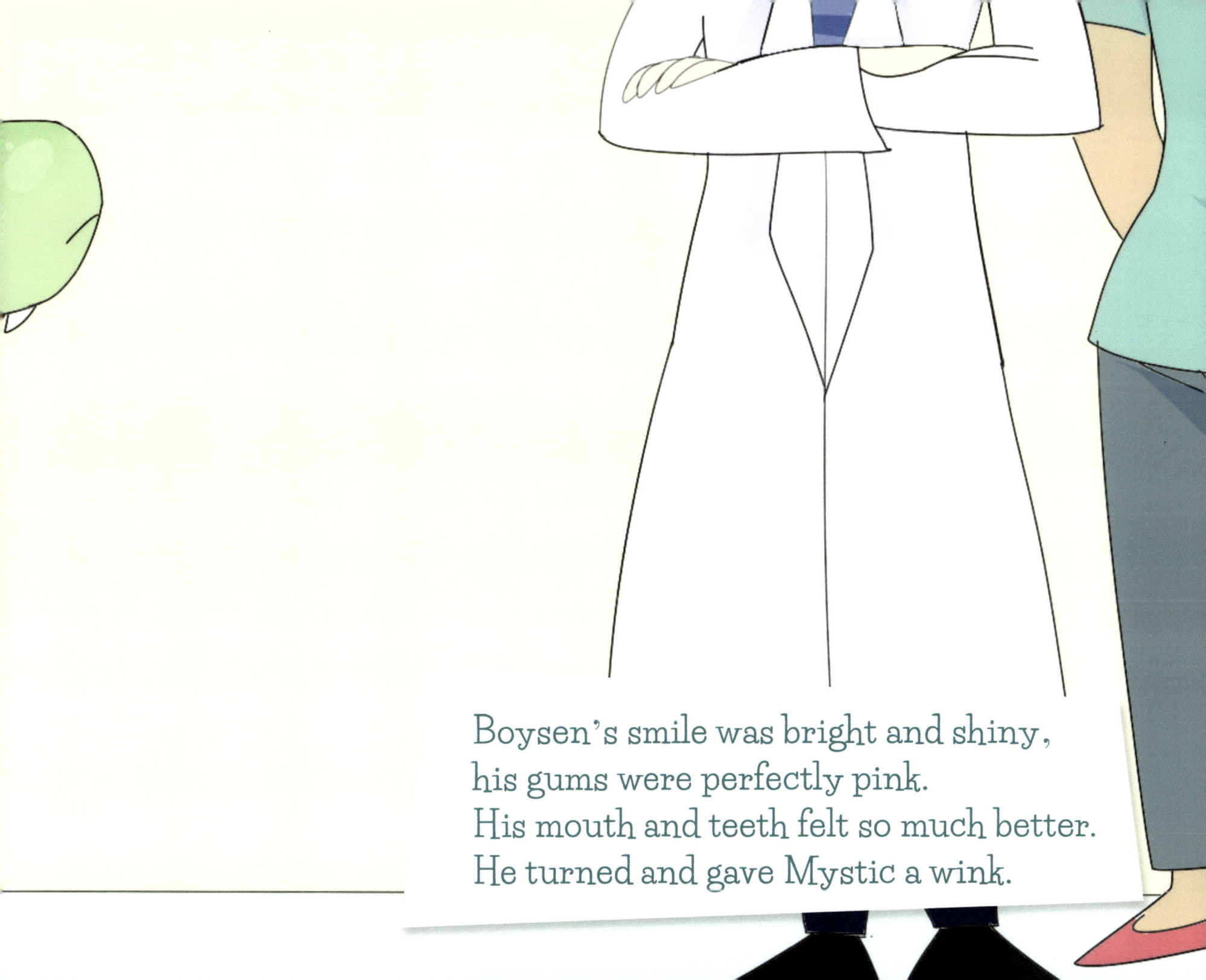

Boysen's smile was bright and shiny,
his gums were perfectly pink.
His mouth and teeth felt so much better.
He turned and gave Mystic a wink.

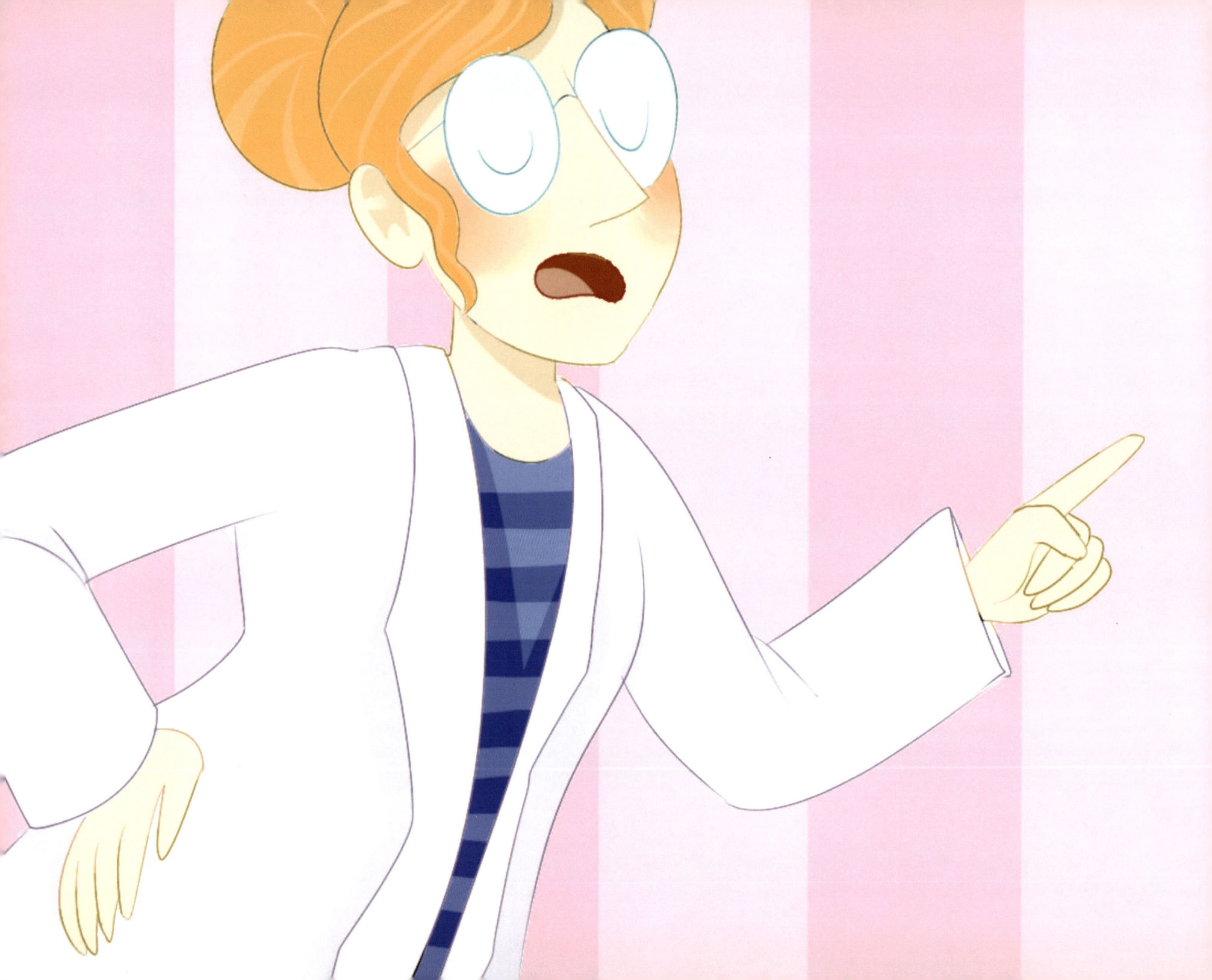

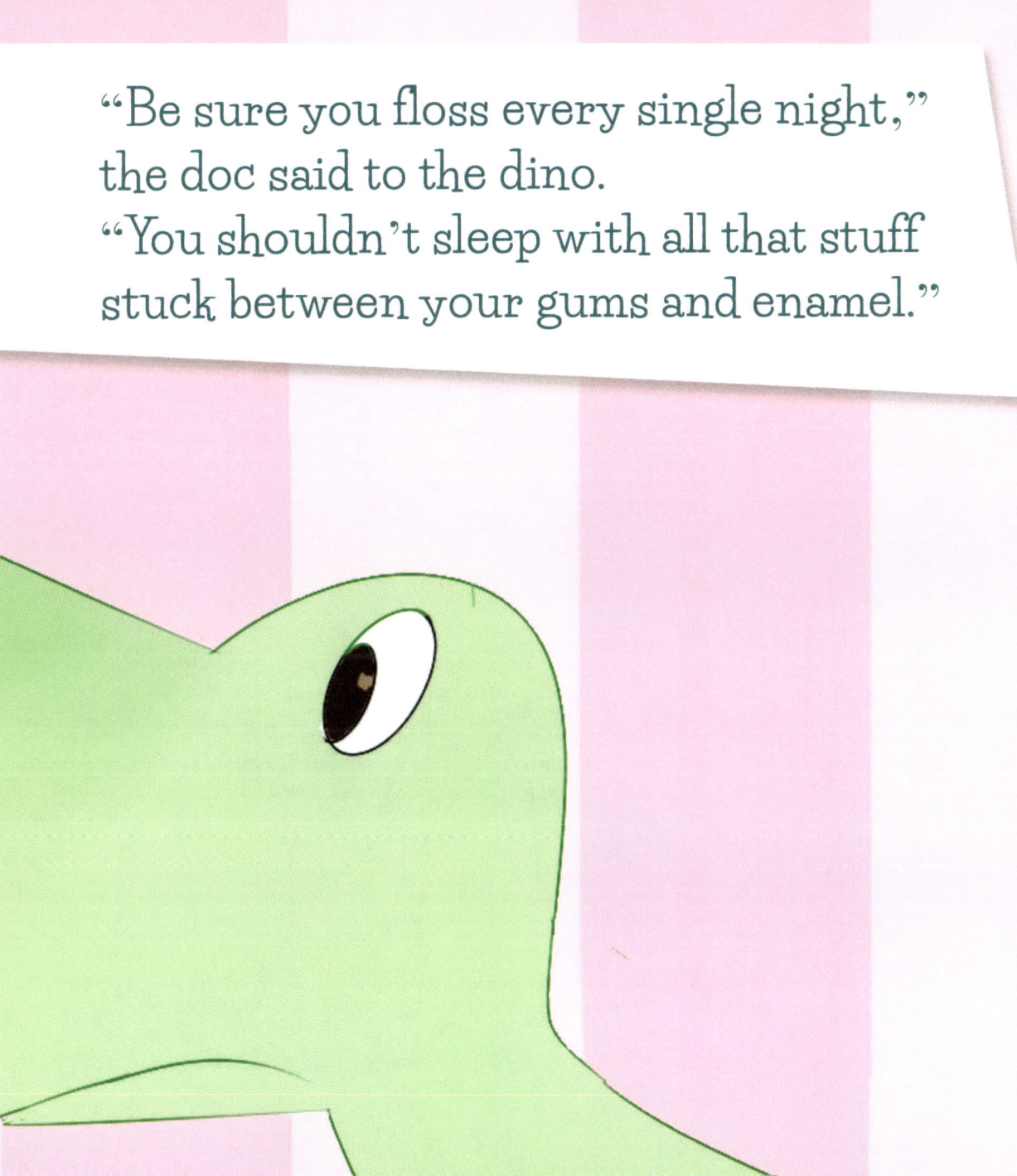

"Be sure you floss every single night,"
the doc said to the dino.
"You shouldn't sleep with all that stuff
stuck between your gums and enamel."

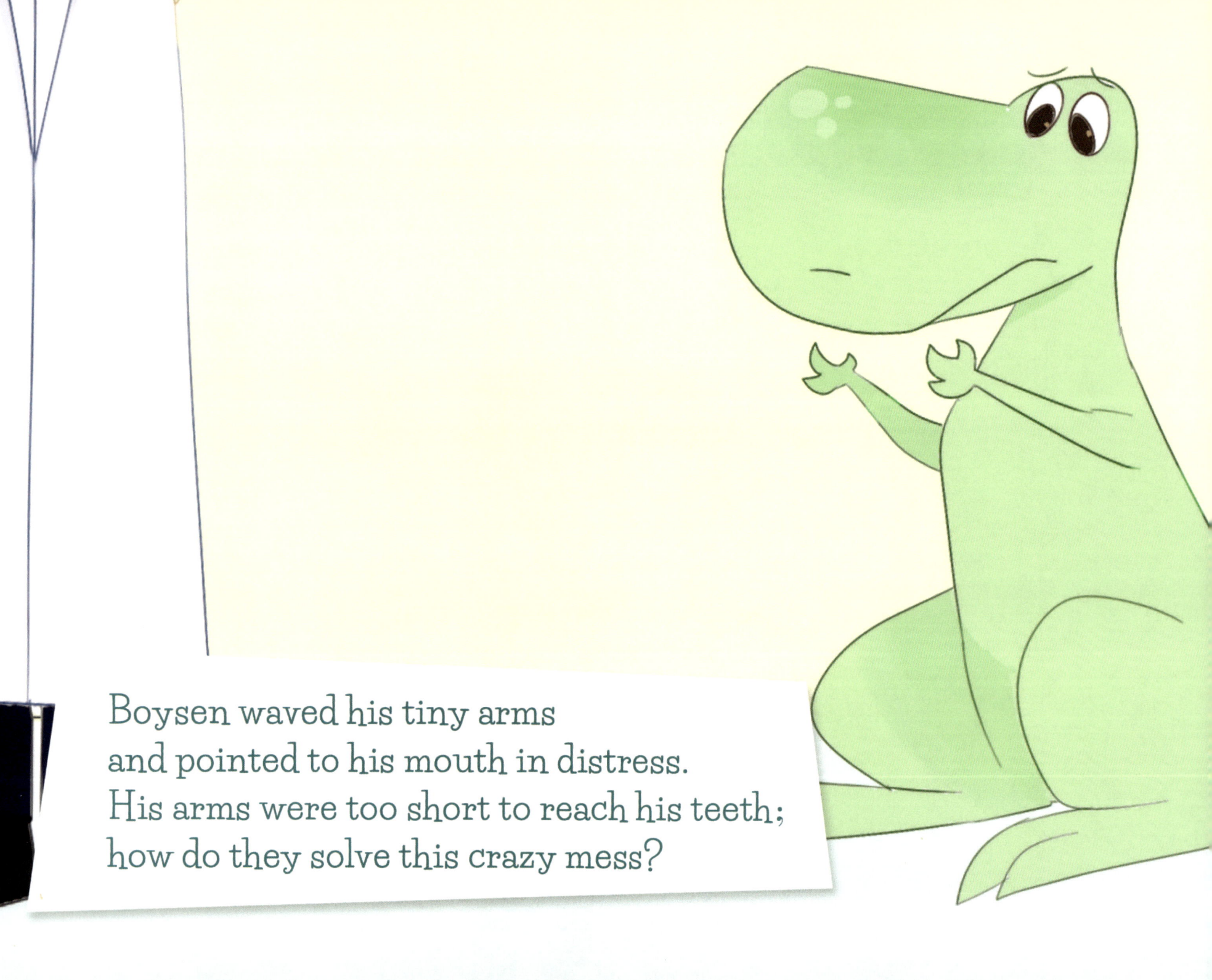

Boysen waved his tiny arms
and pointed to his mouth in distress.
His arms were too short to reach his teeth;
how do they solve this crazy mess?

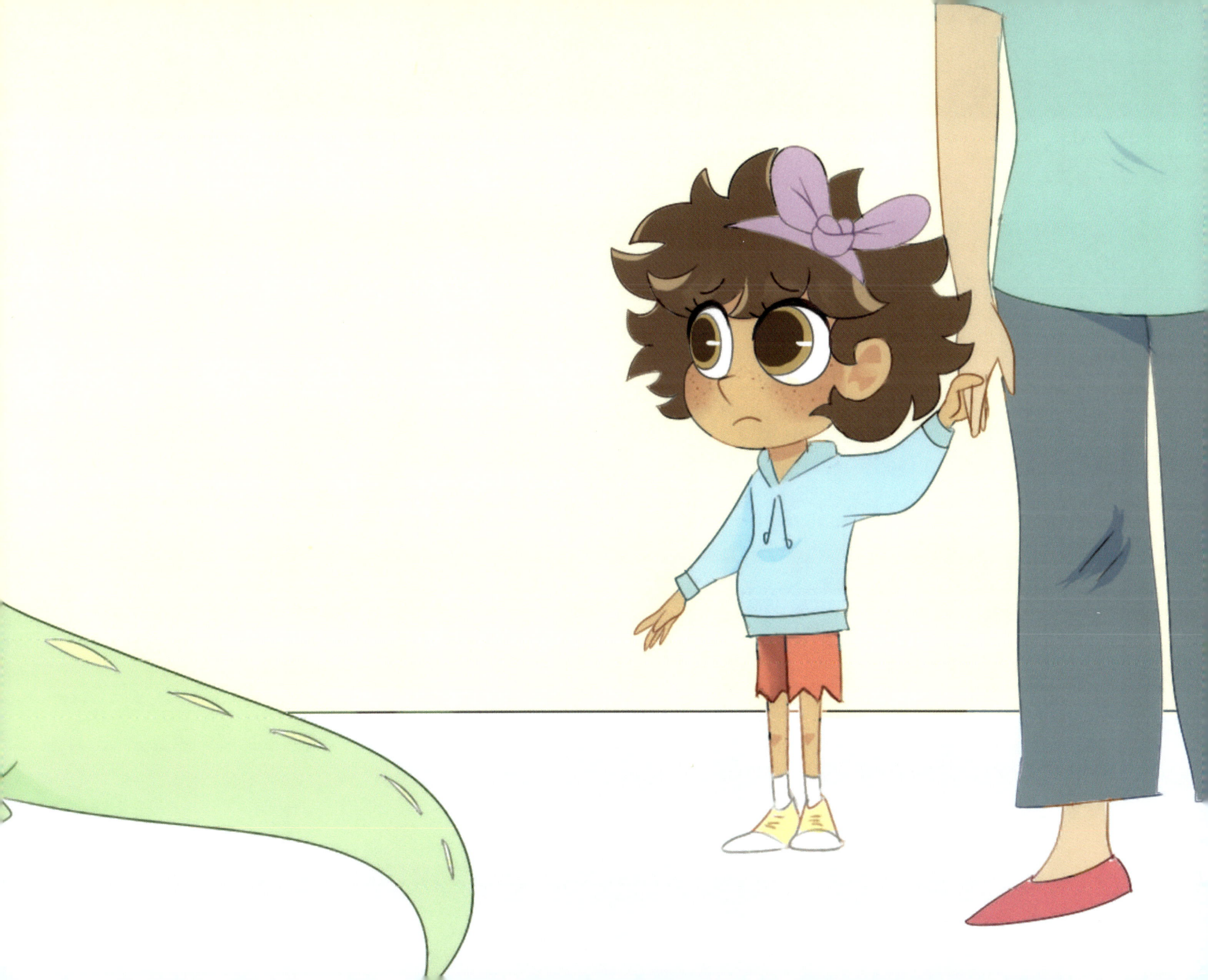

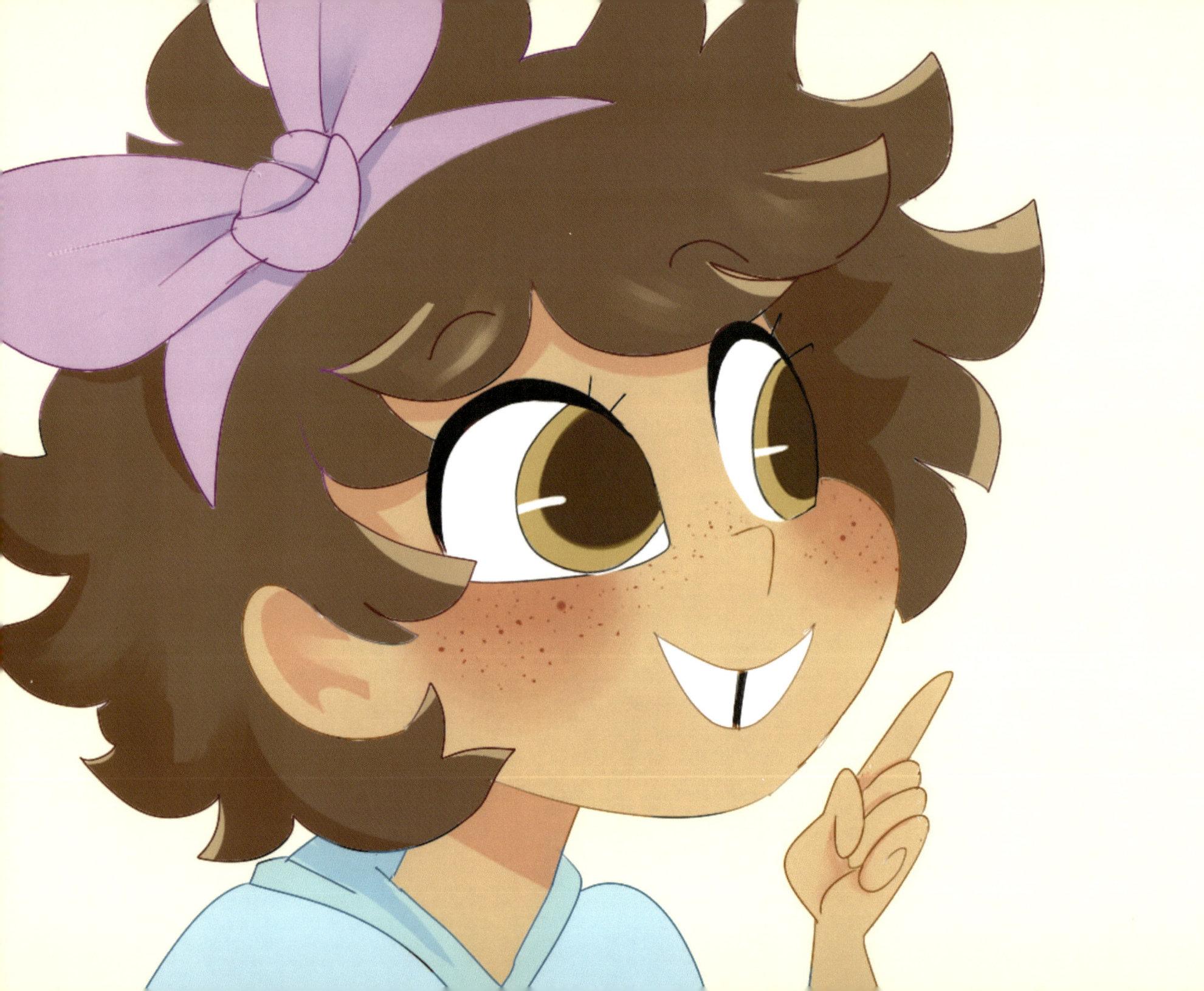

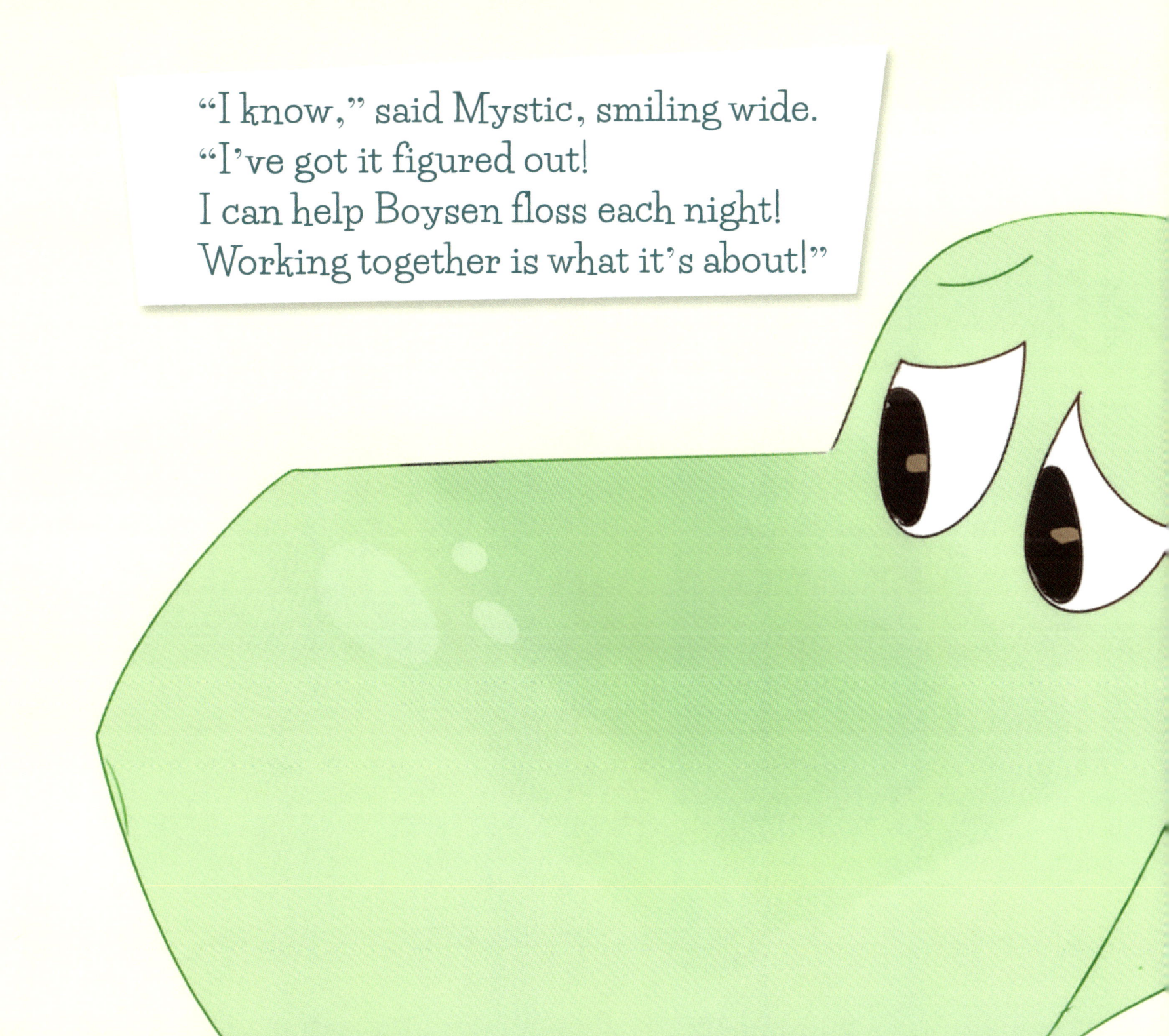

"I know," said Mystic, smiling wide.
"I've got it figured out!
I can help Boysen floss each night!
Working together is what it's about!"

Later that night, Mystic and Boysen
brushed their teeth side by side.
And when it came to flossing two mouths,
Mystic finished the task with pride.

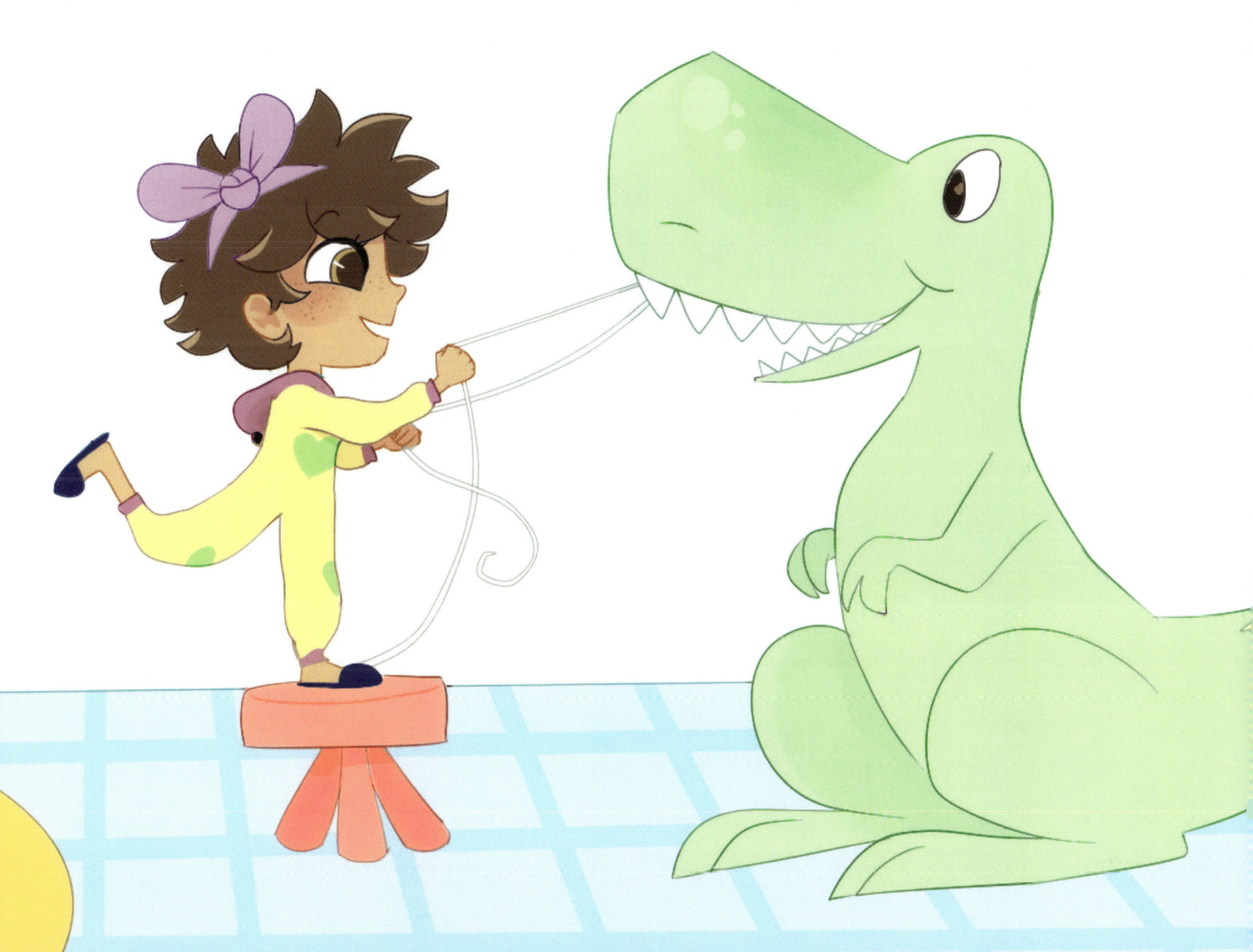

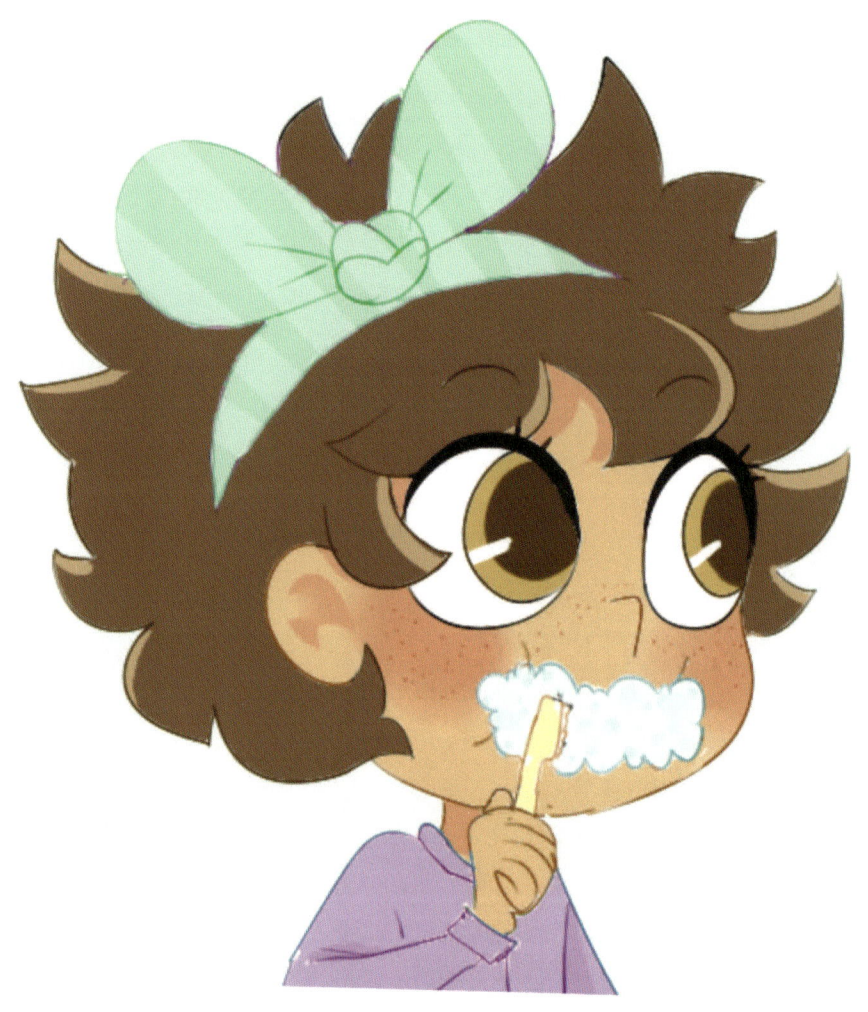

From that day on, and every night,
they brushed and flossed as a team.
This little girl and her dinosaur
work together to keep their mouths clean!

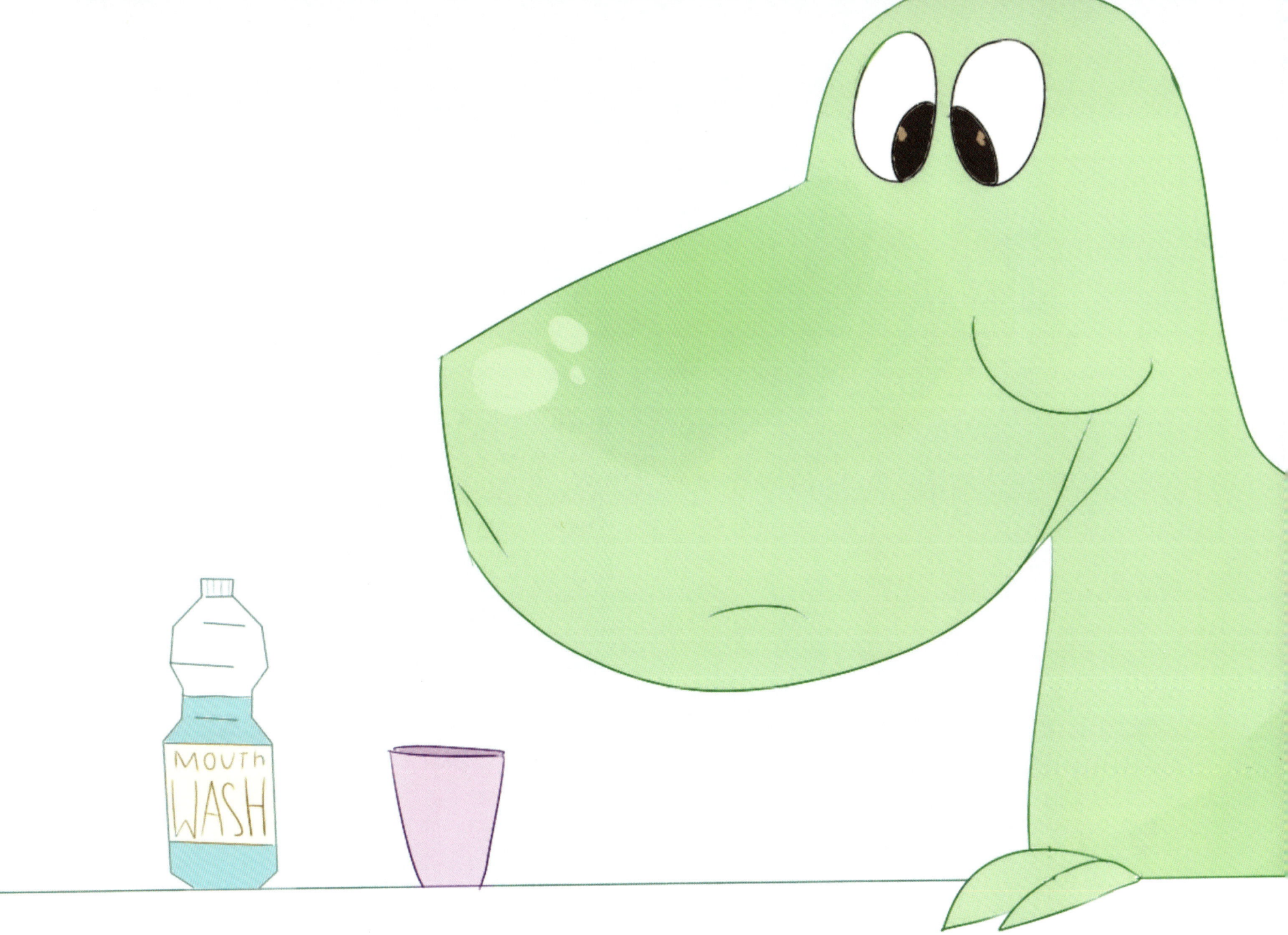

CPSIA information can be obtained at www.ICGtesting.com
Printed in the USA
BVIW121027150819
555974BV00012B/48